FEMALE EJACULATION

FEMALE EJACULATION

UNLEASH THE ULTIMATE G-SPOT ORGASM

BY SOMRAJ POKRAS AND DR. JEFFRE TALLTREES

Amorata Press

Published by: AMORATA PRESS,
an imprint of Ulysses Press
P.O. Box 3440
Berkeley, CA 94703
www.amoratapress.com

ISBN10: 1-56975-679-1
ISBN13: 978-1-56975-679-9
Library of Congress Control Number: 2008928035

Printed in Canada by Transcontinental Printing

10 9 8 7 6 5 4

Acquisitions Editor: Nick Denton-Brown
Managing Editor: Claire Chun
Editor: Melanie Votaw
Proofreader: Abigail Reser
Design and layout: Wade Nights
Cover photo: ©Shutterstock.com/Maksim Shmeljov
Illustrations pages 64 and 71: Derek Aylward

Distributed by Publishers Group West

This book is dedicated to our beloved Tantric family, a continual source of Supreme Bliss through spiritual inspiration, sexual ecstasy, and expanded consciousness.

CONTENTS

CHAPTER 1

INTRODUCTION

"The Constitution only gives people the right to pursue happiness. You have to catch it yourself."

— BEN FRANKLIN

PURPOSES

WHO THIS BOOK IS FOR

If you're reading this book, it's clear that you want to know the depth and breadth of your sexuality. You want to feel great pleasure and amazing sexual ecstasy. You want it all: full-body orgasms, multiple orgasms, extended orgasms with maximum energy that blow your mind, and that elusive and mysterious experience of female ejaculation.

This book is for both men and women. Not only will women learn to achieve female ejaculation, but men will learn how to help women accomplish this little-known sexual phenomenon ... and enjoy the spectacle in the process!

Our goal in creating this book is to show both men and women, opposite sex and same sex couples, how to:

- ♣ Expand your capacity for pleasure.
- ♣ Bring awareness into your sexual play.
- ♣ Routinely reach supreme sexual ecstasy.
- ♣ Build confidence that you can receive and give maximum pleasure.
- ♣ Achieve your full sexual potential.
- ♣ Fully and proudly embrace your sexual birthright.

You'll learn how to awaken that secret orgasmic trigger, the G-spot. You'll learn to give and receive G-spot orgasms of incredible power and sweetness that will ultimately lead to female ejaculation. You'll learn to supercharge your sexual play with the latest scientific findings, discovering a host of new ways to exchange pleasure.

Just as there are many ways to create beautiful music, there are many ways to make love. We're sure you already know how to play some of the instruments in your sexual orchestra. In the coming pages, you'll learn to play those instruments in creative new ways, to play new instruments, and to expand your play list with both.

Soon, you'll become a master of ecstatic alternatives.

But we have to warn you. If you play this tune once, neither of you will ever want to stop.

WOMEN AND ORGASMS

When we started on this path in the mid-1990s, like many women, Jeffre's orgasms required effort. She was never aware of ejaculating. We realized how much we were missing, so we were motivated to learn about pleasure, ecstasy, and orgasm. We've changed so much and had so much fun that we just had to share our journey with courageous, passionate people like you.

So, if you have trouble reaching orgasm during intercourse, you're not alone. Less than half of sexually active women reach orgasm that way. Some estimates claim that 75 percent of women cannot reach orgasm without direct clitoral stimulation. Sadly, 10 to 15 percent of women have never had an orgasm at all. We don't know of any scientific studies that have tracked how many women ejaculate, but we do know that few people seem to be aware of this delightful phenomenon.

You may think you don't have a G-spot. Maybe you haven't been able to find it, awaken it, or stimulate it to orgasm. Maybe you believe you don't or can't ejaculate. But it doesn't have to be that way!

We want you to release your inhibitions, let go of control, and stop holding back. We want you to remember that being alive means feeling intense desire. We want you to know that sexual play is good for you. We want you to celebrate that your orgasms, especially wet ones, make you healthier, more awake, and closer to your lover.

Do you get the idea that we really care about your sex life? You're right, we really, really do.

Unfortunately, most of the so-called civilized world disagrees with our views. We regularly receive referrals from highly trained therapists who are too shy to deal with sexual issues. In fact, too many medical doctors scoff at proven sexual realities like female ejaculation.

This explains why the average lover doesn't know more about their own orgasms.

A SEXUAL HISTORY LESSON

FEMALE EJACULATION'S ANCIENT HISTORY

Is female gushing a new thing? Not in the least. Female ejaculation was well-known and revered in Ancient India thousands of years ago. The Chinese, Japanese, Arabians, Greeks, Africans, Pacific Islanders, and Native Americans all knew about it. Ancient Chinese texts make many references to a woman's "water flowing." Shunga art in 16th century Japan celebrates it in graphic detail.

Western historical references began as early as the 4th century B.C. by Aristotle. Galen, the father of modern medicine, wrote about it in the 2nd century A.D. Interestingly, even William Shakespeare makes reference to "the water of my love."

The first modern description of female ejaculation came in 1672 by the Dutch physiologist, Regnier DeGraaf. He wrote that during the sexual act, the G-spot discharges a fluid so copiously that it even flows outside the vagina. He explained where it comes from and explained that the "rushing out" of this fluid "with impetus" and "in one gush" causes as much pleasure for women as ejaculation does for men.

GIMME A G-SPOT

Where exactly is the G-spot? Generally speaking, it's a highly sensitive area on the front or upper wall of the vagina. The term *G-spot* was coined by Ladas, Whipple, and Perry in their 1982 book, *The G-spot and Other Discoveries About Human Sexuality*. They named the G-spot after Ernst Gräfenberg, M.D., who first wrote about this "new" orgasmic trigger in a scientific journal in 1950.

By the way, Gräfenberg didn't call it a spot—and rightly so. It's an area that exists in different places depending upon the woman. And it moves. Maybe that's why it's often called the "secret orgasmic trigger" and why this doorway to gushing orgasms is an enigma to so many. But this area that we call the G-spot contains the power to unleash hidden emotions, generate deep orgasms, and trigger ejaculation when it is aroused enough. How's that for both complex and powerful?

Though G-spot is a modern term, undoubtedly the ancients were aware of the super-sensitive parts inside the vagina. They were certainly aware of female ejaculation. There are references to the female expulsion of fluid with orgasm as early as the Kama Sutra.

It wasn't until about 400 years ago that a Dutch anatomist, Regnier De Graaf, clearly defined the glands and ducts that make up the G-spot. He said they were analogous to the male prostate. This started a scientific trend of referring to the G-spot as the female prostate.

In 1880, Alexander Skene, M.D. extensively studied and illustrated the glands and ducts that comprise the "female prostate." To this day, some refer to this part of a woman's anatomy as Skene's glands. It wasn't until 1953 that an urologist named Samuel Berkow concluded that this tissue inside the vagina could fill with blood and become erect, similar to a penis or your nipples.

More current research beginning in the 1980s concluded that the Skene's glands are small, functional organs that possess cells comparable to the male prostate gland and secrete similar fluids.

So, when you feel the G-spot, you're feeling these glands beneath the skin of the vagina's upper wall.

MORE RESEARCH, MORE ARGUMENTS

About the turn of the 20th century, Freud was generating his own revolution about the nature of sexuality. He said there were two kinds of female orgasm: clitoral and vaginal. Freud convinced many that clitoral orgasms were immature. According to him, it took a real woman to have a vaginal orgasm.

In contrast, pioneering sex researchers like Kinsey in the 1950s and Masters and Johnson in the 1960s believed that women were only capable of having clitoral orgasms. The good news is that these findings inspired vibrator-wielding feminists to teach women that they could develop their orgasmic potential. The bad news is that many people ignored the G-spot as a valuable source of female sexual pleasure.

Fortunately, the pendulum began to swing back in 1982 when the G-spot book was published. Public consciousness, fueled by scientific research and growing comfort with the sexual revolution, opened to these other orgasmic triggers.

Don't expect your family doctor or even your OB/GYN to know very much about sex. In most medical schools, the training devoted to sexuality is either non-existent or minimal. A few medical schools increased their emphasis on sexuality in the 1970s and 1980s, but many of them have cut back since then. So, it's no surprise that the controversies over the existence of the G-spot, different kinds of orgasms, and female ejaculation continue to this day in the medical community. In fact, the majority of physicians we've met over the years don't accept that female ejaculation is even possible. Of course, we beg to differ!

It's only since the late 1990s that medical researchers began to seriously consider that female sexuality differs from male sexuality. At last, serious investigation into the unique sexual anatomy and physiology of women is under way, and what you will read in this book is based on the most recent findings.

WOMEN ARE DIFFERENT? NO KIDDING!

Yes, male-dominated science finds it difficult to describe female sexuality with simple linear models and reproducible formulas. The fundamental fact that continually appears in our reading, research, and client work is that *every woman is different*. Although there are some general commonalities, each woman has her own inclinations, preferences, and even her own kinds of orgasms.

Your pleasures, sensitivities, and climaxes differ based on factors within and without: your anatomy, hormone levels, mood, level of arousal, connection to your partner, openness to passion, acceptance of her own sexuality, and where you are in your monthly cycle.

But never fear: your G-spot is alive and well and living inside. When you discover exactly what it wants, it can shower you and your lover with delicious peaks of pleasure and sweet female ejaculate.

As our title suggests, female ejaculation is our primary objective here. We're going to prove to you that it's quite common, feels wonderful, and is great to learn. And no, female ejaculate is *not* urine. (In fact, Jeffre had to talk Somraj out of using "tastes great, less filling" here.)

A significant percentage of women already know they gush, squirt, or dribble when they orgasm. Some researchers theorize that all women ejaculate when they orgasm, although for some, this may only be a few drops.

Some women ejaculate only with G-spot stimulation. Others may ejaculate with either G-spot or clitoral stimulation. Some let loose only when both are stimulated. You'll certainly want to play with them all and discover what works for you!

Female ejaculation sounds a little bit clinical, though, doesn't it? We like to keep things simple, but sometimes we just have to use terms that turn us on more. So, we often refer to ejaculating as "letting the waters flow" and female ejaculate fluid as "divine nectar of the receiver." Now, isn't that more exotic and erotic?

HOW TO MAKE THE MOST OF THIS BOOK

SEXUAL EXPLORATION JOURNAL

When Somraj was a chemist, he learned to document everything about scientific experiments in laboratory notebooks. You might want to use a similar approach while reading this book.

To raise self-awareness, many readers find great benefit in recording their thoughts, reactions, and discoveries in a personal journal dedicated to sexual exploration. We suggest you get one right away. Then, as you read this book, you can jot down what you agree with, what makes a strong impact on you, and what doesn't jive with your experience.

When you do the practices sandwiched throughout the book, you're bound to learn a great deal about your body, your sexuality, and yourself. Capturing your adventures offer valuable insight as you progress and help you remember important discoveries. You don't want to have a gushing orgasm only to forget how you got there! Journaling becomes an invaluable tool when you choose to communicate to a lover what you've learned about pleasuring your G-spot.

During all the practices in this training program, we don't expect or encourage complete instant transformation. So, writing down what happened can help you pick up where you left off next time. The G-spot and female ejaculation can even push emotional buttons and raise issues buried deep inside. You'll want to take some breaks to process what comes up, clear the decks, and integrate what dawns on you throughout this process.

To energize your journaling, you'll find discussion questions similar to the following spread throughout the book. You can answer the questions and/or write whatever comes to you. If you're anything like the average couple, talking about sex isn't the easiest thing to do. Those who go through this program with a partner find that these questions are great ways to stimulate honest intimate communication.

EXERCISE: JOURNAL DISCUSSION QUESTIONS

♣ How big is your capacity for pleasure?

♣ How much intimacy and energy do you bring into your loveplay?

♣ What are your orgasms like? Difficult? Full-body? Multiple? Continuous?

♣ How much of your sexual potential do you believe you've realized up to now?

DON'T BE IN A HURRY

Female Ejaculation is full of frank, accurate, up-to-date information about your sexual landscape, including a detailed description of female sexual anatomy. More importantly, we have richly punctuated the pages with hands-on exercises and practices you can use to quickly teach yourself these powerful sexual skills. Along the way, you'll undoubtedly drop negative sexual attitudes, release inhibitions, and awaken dormant responses.

EXERCISE: EJACULATION READINESS CHECKLIST

We've compiled a short checklist for you to fill out so you can find out how ready you are to let those feminine waters flow. Though it's written in the first person, partners can replace "I" with "she" and "my" with "her" to rate their beloved's readiness to ejaculate.

For women, ejaculation is the culmination of everything you'll learn in this book. You can use this checklist as you progress to gauge your progress.

RATING SCALE

To complete the quiz, read each statement, close your eyes, take a deep breath, and feel how much it applies to you. Then score each sentence from 0 to 5 using this rating scale:

5 = Completely describes me all the time.

4 = Mostly describes me.

3 = Sometimes describes me.

2 = Only applies to me a little.

1 = Doesn't apply to me most of the time.

0 = Doesn't apply to me at all, or I don't know if it applies to me.

QUESTIONS

1. I love sex and am entirely proud of it.

2. My attitude is completely sex positive.

3. My mind helps me become totally aroused and romantically engaged.

4. I feel safe and trust my lover, even when my lover is me.

5. I desire to share pleasure and love in my healthy relationship, even when that's with myself.

6. I talk freely and openly about sex.

7. I can relax thoroughly during states of high arousal.

8. I totally love and accept my body and all its parts and fluids.

9. I know all the trigger points that give me the best turn-ons.

10. My tissues and erogenous zones are free and supple.

11. The sexual muscles in my pelvis are strong when I need them and relaxed otherwise.

12. I love my clitoris and know exactly how to please it.

13. I know exactly how to locate my G-spot.

14. I know exactly how to give my G-spot maximum pleasure.

15. I know how to guide a partner to give me maximum pleasure.

16. I show I'm excited by moving, breathing, making sounds, and expressing my emotions.

17. I can easily and reliably reach orgasm.

18. I have multiple, extended, and continuous full-body orgasms.

19. I know how to relax, let go, and push out to ejaculate.

20. I want to shower myself and my beloved with my feminine nectar.

SCORING

Total your scores with a possible maximum of 100. If your total is:

Above 80 — You're ready to go for it.

Between 60 and 80 — You're close.

Between 40 and 60 — You've got some work to do.

But try not to rush it. Orgasms and ejaculation depend on understanding the different kinds of sexual strokes and massage. Stroking depends on understanding anatomy. The further you get in the book, the more we'll refer to earlier concepts and skills.

If you're anything like us, you'll be tempted to skip ahead to the good stuff right away. Since we honor that, we've tried to accommodate you as best we can, but you'll get the most out of the book from reading it start to finish. If you do jump around, we can't promise the techniques will work for you.

Pictures are great. Words are priceless. But it's best if you practice each exercise before moving on to the next one. Whether you're the giver or the receiver, male or female, the more you practice with timely, helpful feedback, the faster and better you'll learn.

Sexual learning is much like working out at the gym, and it relies on the same maxim—use it or lose it. The more you exercise, the easier it gets, and the better it feels. Through practice, you heal the weak parts to make your sexual system healthy and whole.

WHAT'S IN IT FOR YOU

If you've had negative experiences with G-spot stimulation, such as discomfort or a burning sensation, let us assure you that by following our program to awaken your G-spot and female ejaculation, this will never be the case again.

We've created a book that is both comprehensive and user-friendly. In the coming chapters, you will find powerful techniques to master your own sexual forces. You'll learn how to use these techniques to feel the kind of pleasures you have only imagined in your most erotic dreams.

If your score is below 40, you'll want to take every practice in this book very seriously, using them to create a long-term program. The good news is that you have much fun and juicy pleasure awaiting you. We envy you all the growth and self-discovery ahead. You absolutely can expand your sexuality—we're sure of that!

Whatever your score, before you finish reading this book and completing its many juicy practices, you will have learned female anatomy, sexual and massage strokes, and more pathways to G-spot orgasm and female ejaculation than you can imagine.

So, what are you waiting for?

CHAPTER 2

BUILDING ORGASMIC ENERGY

"Ultimately, your definition of sex or sexuality is limited only by your imagination and willingness to explore."
— FROM *HOTTER SEX, DEEPER LOVE* BY JEFFRE TALLTREES AND ORV FRY

LEARNING TO PLAY WITH ORGASMIC ENERGY

WHAT IS ORGASMIC ENERGY?

To experience amazing G-spot orgasms and female ejaculation, a woman must first discover how to master her own sexual energy. By "sexual energy," we mean the subtle, inner vibrations that always percolate beneath most people's consciousness.

Everything in the physical universe is in motion as a result of energy. The cells in our bodies, the blood in our veins, and the impulses in our nerves all continuously vibrate inside because of energy. So, why not our sexual responses and orgasms?

What causes goose bumps? A chill down your spine? Shivers or ticklishness? Or how about that tingly warm feeling in your genitals when you see somebody gorgeous walking down the street. That's sexual energy!

So, when we refer to energy, we're talking about the stimulation and physical excitation that causes these feelings. In China, it's called *chi*. In India, it's called *prana*. In Japan, it's called *ki*, and in yoga, it's called *Kundalini*. But it's all energy. We're talking about the same electrical and magnetic life force that pervades all of our bodies. Because most lovers feel this kind of sexual energy most strongly just before an orgasm, we'll use the term "orgasmic energy." Kundalini is probably the more correct term, but it's all the same electrical or magnetic stuff in your body. Regardless of your level of satisfaction with your lovemaking skills, energy is at the root of it.

To fully enjoy your sexuality and experience the most explosive, gushing orgasms, you need to become aware of these subtler, finer energetic frequencies. Most people don't notice them because their internal receivers haven't been tuned to pick them up. That's partly why we delight in exploring our senses of taste, sight, smell, and sound, as well as a deeper appreciation of sensual touch. By tuning our senses, we learn how to summon orgasmic energy, focus on its effects, magnify its impact, and circulate it around the body, ultimately resulting in a big, wet orgasmic explosion.

EXERCISE: DISCUSSION QUESTIONS FOR WOMEN

- ♣ How are your orgasms? What are they like?

- ♣ Do they come easily? What pushes you over the top?

- ♣ Would you like something more?

- ♣ Do you think you have ever ejaculated?

STREAMING ORGASMIC ENERGY

When enough sexual pleasure is awakened inside, it's hard to contain the orgasmic energy in one spot. So, with any luck, it spreads. People use different words for this: moving, running, channeling, circulating, or streaming energy.

Though they all mean roughly the same thing, *streaming* is probably our favorite term. The name refers to opening your pathways to the energy of ecstasy (even without sexual stimulation) and letting the natural vibrations engulf you. Streaming feels like a flood of pleasure coursing through your body. It's as if every cell is coming. Yes, you feel the same ecstatic experience everywhere. Full-body orgasm is high on our private list of delights!

When we first started practicing energy streaming, Jeffre used to have powerful session-ending orgasms. When she learned to stream instead of explode, she started experiencing multiple orgasms and, eventually, female ejaculation.

When you learn how to stream orgasmic energy when you are by yourself, you can then exchange it with your partner. Contrary to popular belief, the most intense sexual encounters don't result just from sleeping with a really hot woman or skilled man. The pinnacles of sexual ecstasy result from both partners sharing, combining, and building on each other's energy. That's why our definition of S.E.X. is Subtle Energy eXchange.

Why bother learning how to stream?

- ♣ Because it's the key to unleashing the full potential of your sexual power.

- ♣ Because it's how you take yourself higher and higher.

- ♣ Because it's how you learn to awaken your G-spot and the multiple and extended orgasms awaiting you there.

- ♣ Because it's how a woman can build up enough energy to ejaculate.

- ♣ Because it's an amazing feeling!

Some say that women are generally more sensitive to energy and can learn how to stream more easily. Maybe so. But guys can feel it, too. Some can respond intensely to the slightest stimulation with a little practice (which, incidentally, is the secret of overcoming premature ejaculation).

IF INNER TENNIS, WHY NOT INNER ORGASM?

You know what happens to men if all of the sexual energy generated through lovemaking stays in their genitals? When all of this excitement boils over too quickly, the easiest direction for the energy to move is up and out. And then his penis explodes with a momentary flash of pleasure and a big wet spot that usually ends the playtime for a good long while, sometimes leaving his lover unsatisfied.

If he learns how to spread that orgasmic energy away from his genitals and around his body, he'll feel great all over without a sudden big gush. As a result, he can have lots of little energy rushes that get bigger and bigger and bigger, culminating in a long series of internal energy climaxes we call Implosive Orgasm (a process we explain in our previous book, *Male Multiple Orgasm*).

Women can use this same principle of circulating and storing their orgasmic energy in order to build up enough force and pleasure to achieve female ejaculation.

WHERE DO YOU STORE YOUR ENERGY?

Many ancient cultures, both in the East and West, studied our subtle energies and devised methods to gain greater mastery over them. Common to many practices are the *chakras*, the Indian word for wheels. Chakras are whirlpools or vortexes of energy centered at the spinal column and extending in front of and behind the body where subtle energy is generated, collected, and stored.

Most systems identify seven chakras that reside from the bottom of the spine to the top of the head. Here is a relatively universal list:

CHAKRA LOCATION

1st	Perineum; Base of spine
2nd	Belly; 2 inches below navel
3rd	Solar Plexus; Below breast bone
4th	Heart; Center of chest
5th	Throat; Throat
6th	Third Eye; Forehead
7th	Crown; Top of head

Though energy is energy, when it's generated or settles in a specific chakra, it feels different. When we talk about sexual energy, we're actually referring to vibrations of the first two chakras at the belly and pelvic floor. At the heart, it's the warm embrace of love. In the brain, it fuels higher awareness. At the crown, it connects us to the spiritual plane.

All of this may sound foreign to you, but don't worry: you don't have to understand your chakras fully. All you have to do is imagine the energy flowing when the time comes. You don't have to work hard at it, and you don't have to sweat it. Just think of it as play. We're sure you'll be surprised by what you can feel if you practice!

A PRESCRIPTION FOR PROLONGED PEAK EXPERIENCES

So, how do your chakras figure into achieving female ejaculation? First, most love partners want more than just a lust connection. Concentrating on merging the energy of your chakras can be immensely satisfying. You can even use the chakras to move orgasmic energy throughout your body. Doesn't that sound delicious?

Those who practice Kundalini Yoga believe this orgasmic energy sleeps at the base of the spine. Others believe the first chakra resides at the clitoris. Our experience is that the most powerful sexual energies are stored in the G-spot. If you learn to stream sexual energy up and down your chakras, you'll be able to clear the mental, emotional, and physical blocks that stand in the way of an ecstatic sexual experience with your beloved.

STREAMING FOR FUN AND PROFIT

Our biology certainly produces lots of sexual energy, especially when we're young, healthy, or infatuated with a new love. But what happens when you age or get stressed by sickness or life pressures? Then, you can't depend on hormones to turn you on and make you high. If you master running your energy, this will never be a problem. Learn to generate and channel orgasmic energy, and you can reach mind-boggling heights any time you want.

Where do you channel the energy generated? How do you spread it around your body and share it with the one you love? By using your intention, your mind, and your breath, you can learn to send energy anywhere you want.

Move the energy up to the belly, the solar plexus, the heart, the brain, and above. Then it excites, enlivens, and enriches your whole body. That's what makes magic happen and leads to that wonderful fluid from your G-spot. That's why you came to this party, right?

We believe that the G-spot is such a captivating trigger zone because it stores so much orgasmic energy. With a little bit of dedicated practice, you can unleash these powerful forces with even just a small amount of stimulation.

Regardless of your gender, streaming orgasmic energy awakens the rest of your body so that you can experience full-body orgasms. Running energy to the heart awakens your feelings of love and is a powerful turn-on all by itself. Channeling energy to the spiritual centers in the head can make sexual play a transcendent experience.

Once you learn to stream energy, you'll experience amazingly powerful responses to subtle stimuli. Your senses become immeasurably heightened. Imagine what it feels like when other parts of your body are throbbing with the same excitation that makes your genitals pulse and throb?

ENERGY ORGASM

While a normal physical orgasmic release can feel terrific, we like something we call an Energy Orgasm even better. We achieve this by contacting our most powerful trigger zones like the G-spot and generating huge orgasmic energy. Then, we recycle the orgasmic energy rather than expel it. We conserve that energy, and instead of discharging, the energy expands inward, flooding the entire body with pulsing orgasmic contractions and continuous wavelike vibrations.

An energy orgasm is an experience of prolonged peak pleasure in which your whole body vibrates with wave after wave of intense ardor. You shake all over, engulfed in surge after surge of pure liquid fire. And this is when women often ejaculate over and over and over.

Most people experience orgasm from physical stimulation, building up sexual tension and then releasing it. An energy orgasm is an event—a state of ecstasy that's more than just physical, involving many or all of the chakras.

WHERE CAN I GET ONE?

So, how do you experience these delicious energy orgasms? Wouldn't you like to know? And we're going to tell you! Some women get there through stimulation of the clitoris, some get there through intercourse, and some learn to channel orgasmic energy to and from all parts of their body. But we have found that the most powerful access to this zenith of sexual pleasure is through the G-spot.

Many women rarely experience this kind of sexual peak. But when introduced to G-spot play, they report many of the same sensations as we describe for energy orgasm. It just happens naturally! They experience long, continuous pulsing followed by the expulsion of fluid, or they describe it as "going somewhere else and losing touch with reality." It's a wonderful out-of-control feeling that can go on and on and higher and higher.

Is creating the ultimate pleasure worth some delightful practice now and then? You betcha. Once you acquire the knack, you'll never settle day in and day out for "normal sex" again.

EXERCISE: ENERGY ORGASM DISCUSSION QUESTIONS

♣ Have you ever had a full-body orgasm?

♣ Have you ever had an energy orgasm?

♣ Have you ever ejaculated during one of these orgasms?

♣ Have you ever had multiple orgasms of any kind that went on and on?

PRACTICING WITH ORGASMIC ENERGY

THE FOUR CORNERSTONES

Many of you are reading this book not simply to achieve female ejaculation, but to have ecstatic experiences. Along with learning the physical triggers, you'll learn here how to use orgasmic energy to propel you higher and lead you to energy orgasms and ejaculation.

The secret is to turn the responses of the body and mind during orgasmic ecstasy into skills you can practice and master. We call these keys the four cornerstones of Supreme Bliss. They are:

♣ Belly Breathing

♣ Sound

♣ Movement

♣ Presence

The kind of breathing we're talking about is deep, slow, and in the belly. This fuels the body and helps you to make sounds like moaning to express the pleasure you're feeling. This, in turn, releases inhibitions and opens powerful nerve channels.

The kinds of movements we're talking about are undulating pelvic rocking on the outside and sexual muscle pumping on the inside. Not only do these actions channel your energy throughout your body, but they feel really hot, too!

Presence means being relaxed enough to open your senses in the moment without any goal or expectation and focus totally on the pleasure you're feeling *right now*. Presence of mind allows you to use visualization to move your energy, and presence of spirit tunes your internal receiver to the frequency of subtle energy.

INTERNAL TOOLS

These may seem like simple skills, and they are. We're talking about the kind of intense breath, sound, movement, and presence that you usually only experience during an orgasm.

The four cornerstones of supreme bliss consist of the kind of breathing, sound, movement, and presence that happens when you have a typical exciting explosive orgasm. We're going to practice these tools without sexual arousal at first in order to develop mastery over those body/mind functions that happen involuntarily during a climax.

You might think that you already know what turns you on, and usually it's external stimuli. In contrast, the four cornerstones are *internal* tools that you can use to energize your own pleasure and steer your own excitement. If you can learn to use these cornerstones to turn yourself on without external stimuli, imagine what it will feel like when your partner is there?

If you use these cornerstones to consciously get your sexual motor running long before you approach the pinnacle of orgasm, they can empower you to go higher and higher and achieve ejaculation.

For the most part, we'll be dealing here with subtle energies. At first, don't expect that you'll be flipping one of those big high-voltage control levers with huge sparks that will throw your body across the room. To start, although it may take some practice, you'll become aware of a little warmth, electrical tingle, or pleasurable tickle.

It's like learning to tune in to a much higher frequency sound than you're accustomed to hearing, sort of like developing canine hearing. You have to clear your mind and listen acutely to reach it. Once you learn to tune your receiver to subtle sexual energy, it becomes a powerful force. You can direct and regulate it for magnified passion, lighting a long slow burn instead of an overwhelming eruption.

RELAXING

Can you understand how any mental or physical tension can prevent your progress at this stage? You can force your way around solid obstacles with the force of your will. But to use subtle energy, you have to relax, breathe, and feel every little sensation. Tension will block the doorway to feeling and moving these energies. It may feel more like an experience of *allowing* the flow of energy.

Don't worry about how fast you go, and never despair when it takes longer than you'd like. Soon, you'll get inklings, followed by surges, and finally culminating in waves that will bowl you over, leading to the ejaculation you're after. Be patient. You'll probably need to practice numerous times for several weeks before the magic will occur. Somraj took months before he could feel orgasmic energy and move it. Take it easy with yourself and your partner.

BELLY BREATHING

Most of us take breathing for granted, and we tend to take shallow and unconscious breaths. Contrast that with yoga masters. Some are so aware of their breathing that they can shut it down to almost nothing and stay in a state of suspended animation for extended periods.

Remember what happens to your breath as you approach orgasm? Right, your breath becomes shorter and faster, and you may even pant uncontrollably.

We could all benefit from mastering the art of belly breathing, which is characterized as follows:

- ♣ Relaxed
- ♣ Through the mouth
- ♣ Deep in the belly.

This kind of full breathing lowers your heart rate and dissipates the tension of arousal. Breathing through your mouth is more physical and sensual as opposed to breathing through your nose, which tends to put your attention in your mind.

So, one of the best ways to relax when you're excited is to learn to breathe slower and deeper. It helps to interrupt the stress response you may experience during exciting or anxious moments of lovemaking.

Belly breathing is such a basic part of running energy that we could go on and on about going slow and savoring the experience. Actually, a great way to learn how to do a belly breath is to recognize that it has four parts:

- ♣ In
- ♣ Pause
- ♣ Out
- ♣ Pause.

We're not talking about holding your breath as long as you can, but simply not rushing ahead to the next in or out. Simply pause for a distinct moment between inhaling and exhaling, exhaling and inhaling, so that you can notice how you're feeling.

MAKING SOUNDS

Next, you have a chance to practice one of the most powerful of the four cornerstones: sound.

- ♣ Do you moan at all during lovemaking?
- ♣ Does it make you feel self-conscious?
- ♣ How about when you're coming?

Sound is one of the most powerful cornerstones of ecstasy. The same nerves that regulate your voice box are connected to your sex organs. When your orgasmic reflexes are working, moaning with pleasure comes naturally. In fact, it requires more energy to repress your voice. If you didn't stop yourself, you'd have that much more energy to fuel your passion!

So, the more noise you make, the more passionate you'll feel inside. The more passionate you feel inside, the more passionate you'll appear. And guess what, the more passionate you appear, the more you'll feel inside, and the more likely you'll experience an energy orgasm and ejaculation. It's a self-reinforcing loop.

Just remind yourself that pleasure is your divine birthright, and you're entitled to as much ecstasy as you can conjure up. Sounding off is one way to amplify your sensations. If you're in the least self-conscious about being overheard, be sure to find a quiet place where no one can hear you no matter how loud you become.

VISUALIZING ENERGY

Next, we're going to add the visualization of energy along with your breathing, pumping, and sounding. Since energy flows where attention goes, just imagining sexual energy and electricity somewhere in your body will make something happen eventually. You already knew that the mind was the most powerful sex organ, right?

We're going to begin working with your chakras in a big way. These are the vortices where energy tends to collect and swirl around at different places inside your body. There is also an energy channel near your spine that connects your chakras. We call this your "inner flute."

Remember to keep all of your senses open. If you feel any sensations, no matter how subtle, visualize your breath passing through the area where you feel the sensations. In this way, the breath adds fuel to a small fire, causing it to flare up with higher flames. Even if you don't feel much, pretend that you do, and breathe into the body parts you want to energize.

PELVIC ROCKING

The four cornerstones of Supreme Bliss include movement. Pelvic Rocking is a rotation of your pelvic area. Some have likened it to riding a horse, but we prefer to compare it to slow deep sexual union when you're on top.

With your weight on your knees and hands over your lover, the only way you can penetrate deeply is by either doing push-ups or by rocking your pelvis forwards and backwards. The latter is what we're adding to your repertoire here.

FLEX YOUR SEXUAL MUSCLES

PC MUSCLE

We want you to start learning to run sexual energy with one aspect of the movement cornerstone, flexing your inner sexual muscles. We're talking about your PC muscle, short for *pubococcygeus*.

We realize that's a mouthful of a medical term, but it's easy to identify. Put one of your hands on your pubic bone, the inside one that's above your genitals and around your pubic hair at the bottom of your tummy. That's the "P."

Now, reach around behind you, and put your other hand near the top of your crack just below your spine. That's your tailbone or coccyx, which is the "C." The PC muscle snakes down around your genitals and anus and connects these two bones plus your sitting bones and legs.

What's more important, you need to be able to identify the PC muscle from the inside. It's the one you tighten when you want to squeeze out the last few drops of urine. Try squeezing it now. Did you feel it?

If you can't isolate it, take a break and go the bathroom right now. Start peeing, and stop in the middle. When you're finished, try to squeeze the last few drops out. The muscle you used to stop midstream and squeeze at the end is your PC muscle.

STRENGTHEN YOUR PC

Having strong internal pelvic muscles, keeping them relaxed when at rest, and knowing how to use them without strain can dramatically enhance your sexual pleasure. Why? Because the PC pulses rhythmically during intercourse, especially strongly during climax as it pumps sexual energy. If your PC muscle is weak, your pleasure and orgasms will suffer. If the muscle is always tense, it can block your ability to stream orgasmic energy.

Did we mention which muscle is primarily responsible for female ejaculation? You've got it: the PC muscle.

If yours is strong, you have a powerful tool to consciously channel energy throughout your whole body. The stronger this muscle becomes, the more intense and pleasurable sexual intimacy can be for you, and the more easily you can have an energy orgasm and ejaculate.

As with any physical exercise, improved tone gives you better muscle control. When a muscle is weak, it feels like mush even after a few contractions. With a weak PC, this cuts off the flow of pleasure and the length of orgasm. When a PC muscle is well-toned, it can relax more easily, and you can continue pumping as long as you want, extending orgasm.

PC PUMPS

Did we convince you that you need to do PC pumps? That's what we call these sexual muscle squeeze practices. Fortunately, it's easy and inexpensive to strengthen them. It just takes a few minutes a day, although it doesn't happen overnight. To get the maximum benefits, we urge you to add some of the following practices to your daily routine.

By the way, you've probably heard of Kegels. These are similar practices developed by a gynecologist in 1952 named Dr. Arnold Kegel. He taught women to strengthen their PC muscles after the trauma of childbirth to restore tone and regain control of their urinary reflexes.

Doing PC pumps is easy. The hard part is establishing a regimen and remembering to do them. Develop a successful memory device so that you don't forget. Find a time and place where you'll remember to do several sets of these practices each day. Once they get strong after months of practice, continue the same regimen as a maintenance program.

You might use the beginning of your commute to and from work as you stop for traffic lights, when you check your email, during TV commercials, in the bathtub, or when you start your workout at the gym.

Whatever you choose, do it regularly so it becomes an integral part of your life routine. Since it doesn't seem to matter what position you're in for these practices, you can choose whenever and wherever best jogs your memory.

Remember, don't push yourself and strain your groin at the outset. Instead, build up gradually. Relax everything else when you do PC pumps. If you tend to tense up, put your tongue on your upper palate to prevent clenching your jaw.

When you start practicing as described in the upcoming pages, you may find that you're also tightening your stomach muscles. Don't worry about it for now. Within a few days or weeks, you'll learn to isolate your muscle control, so that only the pelvic floor where the PC muscle resides will be flexed.

These practices may be about squeezing your PC muscle, but the relaxing in between each contraction is vital. If you're tense, your sexual energy gets trapped and can't flow. So, the unflexed moments between pumps are as important as the strengthening. Get into the habit of squeezing to tone the muscles, but put as much attention on totally relaxing between flexes.

PC EXERCISES

Here's a series of four exercises you can use to strengthen your PC muscles...

PC FLEX

Squeeze and release your PC muscle at the rate of your heartbeat, which means hold it each time for about a second. Start with 20 contractions twice a day, and build up to at least 75 per set. When you can easily do 75 contractions twice a day, add the PC Clench.

PC CLENCH

Practice clenching your PC while inhaling. By clenches, we mean holding the squeeze for a longer period of time. Some experts say 3 seconds, some say 6, some say 15. Maybe they're all correct, so we suggest you start with 3 and work up to 15 seconds per clench.

To do clenches, inhale and clench your PC, holding it tightly. Then, push out and relax for the same amount of time before your next clench. Repeat this cycle 20 times twice a day at first. As with flexes, build up to 75 reps twice a day.

For women, it's very important to spend time on the push-out. Use the instructions above, and inhale, push out, hold for 3-6 seconds. Do the push-out variation of the clench as many times as the pulling-in.

PC FLUTTERS

This practice is basically the same as the first one (PC Flexes), except it's faster. To do flutters, you contract and relax your PC as fast as you can. At first, you may not be able to go much faster than your heartbeat, but with practice, you can speed up the squeeze and release. We suggest you don't count these but just work up to fluttering for several normal breaths before relaxing totally. Doing 20 sets of these twice a day should be great. When you can flutter like a bird, add PC Clamps.

PC CLAMPS

PC Clamps are simply long clenches. Work up to holding your clench for two minutes, 20 times each set. Remember to relax completely at length between these long clamps, and stop for a few minutes if you start to hurt or get sore.

PC practices can be a very intensive regimen if you go full out. So, don't forget to start slow! Once you develop strength and tone in your PC muscle through some weeks of practice, you can back off to a maintenance level of exercises. After a couple of years of intense practice, we don't do every exercise every day. Eventually, you'll develop a sense of what's right for you to make your PC strong and keep it there.

PRACTICE: PRACTICING ORGASMIC BREATHING

Now, let's combine all of the elements of supreme bliss into one comfortable unified whole. We've broken down the individual parts of the four cornerstones of supreme bliss into discreet steps. When we're working privately with clients, we guide them to practice each one separately. But once you learn to coordinate them all, orgasmic breathing is just doing one unified thing. Most people do these things naturally together during ecstatic sex, so why not use them consciously?

1. POSITION

Use whatever position you want as long as it allows free pelvic movement.

2. RELAXING

Spend a few minutes getting comfortable, watching your breath, and releasing any muscle tension. Keep your eyes closed.

3. BELLY BREATHING

Start taking belly breaths.

4. ROCKING

Rock your pelvis one way on the in-breath and the other on the out-breath.

5. PC PUMP

Add the PC pump exercise on the in-breath.

6. SOUNDS

Make sounds as you start to feel good.

7. VISUALIZE

Visualize the energy coming into your first chakra and streaming up your inner flute by the force of your PC contractions. During your first practices, aim to raise your sexual energy just up to your heart chakra. Of course, you can practice moving the energy up to any chakra, all the way to the crown of the head, so do what feels best in the moment.

8. ENJOY

Enjoy the sensations you feel for a few minutes.

9. SYNCHRONIZE

If you want, try this with a partner. Sit across from each with your eyes closed as you perform the first eight steps. When you feel you're in the flow of the energy, open you eyes. When the second partner opens their eyes, coordinate your breathing in and out together at the same pace. Can you feel each other's energy?

AFTERTHOUGHTS

You may have to practice a few times to get the pieces working together. Once you do, just practice this combined exercise several times a week for a few weeks for about 15 minutes each time.

Orgasmic breathing is the primary method of channeling energy when you're making love. It may require repeated practice because at first, it's a very subtle experience for most people. Once you get it, though, it makes for very exciting love play. It sure gets our juices flowing when we do it before sex.

As you continue with this book, you'll find lots of chances to practice as you discover more triggers for female ejaculation.

CHAPTER 3

THE ART OF LOVEPLAY

"You can discover more about a person in an hour of play than in a year of conversation."

— PLATO

START WITH INTIMACY

WHAT IS LOVEPLAY?

Why do we say "loveplay" instead of "foreplay"? The word *foreplay* implies something that you do before the main event. The further implication is that it's of lesser value. But the truth is that any sensation can be the catalyst for a huge flow of passion all by itself. When your energy channels are open, you can circulate and exchange the forces of orgasm even without genital stimulation. When we do experience orgasm from physical stimulation, it's often a continuous rising experience without an explosive crescendo.

This means that "before" and "after" lose their relevance. So, don't establish goals, set expectations, or plan a detailed agenda for your loveplay. Instead, experiment with impulses and fantasies that strike you as fun in the moment. Be playful, spontaneous, and enjoy the journey.

From the moment you begin to change the feel of the space around you, you are being sexual. You are using erotic, orgasmic energy. The instant your eyes meet those of your lover's, you feel tingly inside. The first touch is electric, sending chills and shivers throughout your being. As you honor your beloved and offer thanks for being with you at this time, tears may spring to your eyes. You may feel a strong stirring between your legs long before you take your clothes off.

This is loveplay. We urge you to not miss a single tingle, a tiny shiver, or the subtlest energy surge. This is surely as much sex as anything else you'll ever do.

JUICY THINGS AHEAD

If you're like most women, you'll probably enjoy G-spot play only after an extended warm-up. It's a kind of tissue that swells with arousal, so you may not even feel your G-spot at first, let alone ejaculate.

One study found that the average length of loveplay was 15 minutes, and the average length of intercourse was just 10 minutes. We're well aware that, for maximum enjoyment, the average woman requires 35 to 45 minutes of erotic warm-up to get her juices flowing adequately.

This means that the average lover stops 10 to 20 minutes short of peak female pleasure (which makes us really worry about the less than average lovers). Maybe now, you can understand why there's a dearth of orgasms in the world.

So, this chapter is about experimenting with a wide array of sensitive, sensual, sexual tips to get you both turned on. It's all about pleasure and preparing you for that gushingly wet orgasm called female ejaculation. Though we'll delve into touching, kissing, and licking, you'll find as much emphasis on opening your hearts, tuning your senses, and connecting your feelings. That's because the keys are presence, consciousness, and energy flow, not simply technique. That's what will lead you to experience ejaculation — not just performing step one followed by step two and so on.

WOMEN LOVE WORDS FROM THE HEART

It's often said that women get turned on in the heart first and in the genitals later, while men are just the opposite. When men get turned on in the genitals, that energy moves to the heart.

Although there are always exceptions to this kind of blanket generalization, we believe it's safe to assume that most women, most of the time, like to have their minds and hearts stimulated in the 24 to 48 hours before the actual "date."

Jeffre says it turns her on when Somraj says "I love you." Many women feel this way. A woman may need to ask her man to let her know how much he cares for her, thinks about her, and how much he's looking forward to time alone with her.

Women respond very positively to words and touch that convey feelings of love and affection. Women seem to like words about love, sex, and relationship and feel they're very important. Often, men don't have feelings as strong as women about verbalizations of love.

If you're a guy who feels uncomfortable with words, we humbly suggest that you practice — a lot. Nothing will get you more of what you want than being able to verbalize feelings of affection for your woman. Read a book or two, and write out what you want to say. Practice letting the words tumble over your tongue and lips. Now, say it out loud to your partner. Try something like this: "Honey, I'm having trouble concentrating at work. My heart is swelling with thoughts about your soft skin, your bright eyes, your sweet scent. Please don't be wearing much when I get home early."

By the way, Ladies, guys like romantic words like this as well.

INTIMACY IS A TURN-ON FOR WOMEN

Intimacy is the emotional closeness that truth-telling and feeling loved can bring. For most women, it heightens their turn-on when a man talks about his feelings with honesty and heartfelt expression instead of blame or judgment.

Intimacy can also be about sharing fantasies and playing them out. Often, the fantasies lurking inside are pretty kinky, so lovers can feel uncomfortable sharing them with their beloved. But getting past this inhibition is exciting on multiple levels. The truth-telling is a turn-on because of the increased sense of closeness. Plus, the content of most fantasies can really get your sexual motor going big time. Of course, if your lover's fantasy is a turn-*off* to you, don't pretend that it gets you going, but don't judge it either. Simply keep looking for a fantasy that you both love.

PRACTICE: INTIMACY COMMUNICATION

Women tend to enjoy 30 to 60 minutes of loveplay, while men may request and desire less. Only you can know how your body responds and what feels best.

This practice asks you to discuss, as specifically as possible, the types of loveplay you like and the amount of time you like it. Go over the following questions separately, and share your answers. Let the dialogue flow until you both feel heard and understood.

By the way, this is a starting place. As you become more practiced in these ways, you may want three to six hours of loveplay. Who knows how far you'll go?

1. COMFORT

Do I give or receive most comfortably?

2. PRACTICE

I would like to practice receiving (or giving) more...

3. HONESTY

Sometimes, I'm not honest with you about what I really want. Here's an example...

4. TIME

The amount of time I usually like to spend in loveplay is...

5. KINDS

The kinds of loveplay I like best include...(touching, massage, kissing, talking, fellatio, cunnilingus, etc.)

CHOOSE THE MOOD YOU WANT

One wonderful way to accentuate the sanctity of your love and the consciousness of your underlying passion is how you disrobe. Slowly remove each other's clothing one little piece at a time while caressing, nuzzling, and whispering sweet endearments to each new morsel of flesh that is uncovered.

Perhaps you'll want to bathe together. After a day of busy life activity, this is a wonderful transition to a more sensual mood. Bathe, soap, rub, and slide with each other. Flirt and tantalize with all your parts: lips, eyes, fingers, tongue, breasts, genitals, and any other part of your body that wants to join in. This is how you create heaven on earth.

Spend some time unwinding by just being together. Look deeply into each other's eyes. Synchronize your breathing. Reach out with your consciousness to feel your beloved's energy.

A practice that we do often is called the melting hug. You slowly come closer together until your first contact. Then you melt your bodies into each other with as much skin touching as possible. Relax and cling to each other. Let your breathing synchronize. Feel the connection of your chakras.

KISSING AS AN ART FORM

Kissing is a wonderful form of loveplay because it stimulates so many different energy centers. It's a sweet expression of affection that connects with the heart. Your vision, mind, and third eye are totally focused on your lover. It turns many lovers on with resulting hardness and wetness that encourages the mood for heavier exchange.

Kissing all parts of the body can be divine play. Try lightly kissing your partner's chakras beginning with the 7th (at the top of the head) and ending with the 1st (the perineum.)

AWAKENING YOUR BELOVED'S SENSES

Orgasmic energy is all about staying in the body, opening the senses, and feeling the ecstasy. There are many ways to increase awareness of your body and open the senses. You can dance. You can eat sensual foods. You can walk in the forest. You can meditate.

You can blindfold your beloved and titillate them with tastes, smells, touch, and sounds. Then you can remove the blindfold, and offer glorious sights as you slowly and sensuously reveal your naked body.

Ever tried acting out a silent fantasy in front of your lover? How about pleasuring yourself while your lover is tied down?

The range of possibilities for building anticipation is enormous. Use your imagination, and surprise your beloved. Your loveplay will never get old or stale.

EXERCISE: MOOD DISCUSSION QUESTIONS

- I plan to do the following to create a sacred space before we make love...

- Here's how I intend to heighten intimacy and connection during our loveplay...

- Here's how I'll experiment with awakening my beloved's senses...

TALKING ABOUT SEX

EXCHANGING INFORMATION

We already discussed communication when we prescribed titillation, flirtation, and intimacy. Communication is also essential for exchanging information so that you can enhance your own and your partner's pleasure.

Learning to talk with your partner about sex requires guts and practice. Sometimes, women want to protect their man's ego, and this makes them too polite. Often, they're unsure if they even have the right to ask for anything other than what they're getting. Too many men don't know how, why, or when they want something different.

It's great to create an intention together to be able to talk about sex openly and honestly. Talk about your fears. This is a major frontier for most couples.

That's partly why we urge you to talk before during, and after each practice and lovemaking encounter no matter how long you've been together. Don't worry if you feel you're not eloquent at first. Whatever you do is good for intimacy and will help your communication skills to grow.

It can be helpful to coach or redirect your partner while you're physically intimate. If you make an agreement beforehand about how you want to communicate during sex, it can be much less challenging.

No one likes to feel criticized or put down, most particularly while in bed with a lover.

Hopefully, you're taking advantage of the discussion questions we've included after each major section. These are primarily designed to encourage this whole process of talking freely about sex. After reading, think back about your reactions, write your answers to the questions, and share with your partner. Gradually, you'll transform the intimacy of your connection and create the foundation to transmute subtle energy into awesome ecstasy.

BE REAL

The single biggest communication foul-up is when one or both partners aren't completely forthcoming and authentic with each other. In less formal words, this means acting phony. Of course, when you speak, it's important to be loving and gentle with your words, rather than accusatory or judgmental.

Do you:

- ♣ Feel that your beloved is responsible for satisfying you in any way?

- ♣ Believe that your partner is supposed to automatically know how to satisfy you?

- ♣ Act passive when you're not getting what you want and then, complain afterwards?

- ♣ Wait for that magical moment when something outside of yourself will sweep you away?

The truth is that whether you're female or male, you're 100% totally responsible for your own arousal and orgasms. Of course, we don't mean that all good lovin' is self-lovin', but great sex is a dance in which it takes two to tango.

There are still too many men who think they're failures if their women don't have an orgasm. There are too many women who don't have a clue what will make them feel the ultimate in sexual pleasure. No matter how much you have to learn about your subtle orgasmic triggers and keys to ecstasy, the more you talk with your partner about what you want, the quicker you'll both learn what you can do to get it.

♣ I feel these sexual needs are understood and appreciated...

♣ I want my beloved to better understand...

♣ I feel shy or embarrassed talking about...

COMMUNICATE, COMMUNICATE, COMMUNICATE

As a marriage counselor for many years, Jeffre has learned that the single biggest reason women get turned off to sex (after religion) is their fear of telling their men the truth about their sexual responses, desires, and wants. If you want to deepen and supercharge your sex life, communication must begin at the beginning. That's where the following practice, How To Touch Me, picks up — at the beginning.

Going deeper with communication throughout your loveplay helps tremendously to create intimacy as well. When receiving, women need to explain what they desire, what they feel, and how they're reacting. Although this is true of men too, our focus right now is on preparing women for female ejaculation.

Partners in general, and men in particular, do not appreciate being in the dark (figuratively, of course) when they're trying to please you. They need and want to feel confident that they're successfully turning you on.

Women are not only different from each other, but they're different from one moment to the other. This is confusing to the average guy who's always trying to learn what women want. You'll be better off if you just accept these observations as fact:

♣ No two women's sexual response is identical.

♣ Women like variety — different things at different times.

♣ Hormones change at different times of the month, which can alter a woman's sexual response.

♣ Emotional beings like women have unpredictable moods, which can also alter sexual response.

♣ Sensitive bodies, like female ones, may respond strongly to stress, exercise, medication, health challenges, and menopause.

Okay, guys, you've been warned. Assume nothing!

SPEAK UP AND ENJOY

Are you familiar with that common mental refrain "Am I doing it right?" or the verbal one, "Did you come yet?" These worries stem from self-consciousness and concern about your own sexual performance.

But if you enter into sex without expectations, any such performance anxiety disappears. Your sex becomes a conscious dance of energies, and no longer will you have to worry about what's happening with your partner and if he/she is enjoying your touch. It's like synchronized swimming with telepathic communication.

Good lovers know that they're each responsible for their own plea-sure. They recognize that erotic experiences begin within. They know what they like, what they prefer in the moment, and what to pass on during each encounter. They've explored all pleasure triggers and know when and how they want to be stimulated. They ask for what they want, voice their reactions, and give lots of feedback. And they do it in a way that enhances intimacy and contributes to the sensual mood.

Obviously, this kind of authentic interplay requires knowing, accept-ing, and loving yourself fully. Then you can be completely honest, totally real, and refreshingly transparent with your innermost desires—which leads to knowing, accepting, and loving your partner. And this is the sort of intimacy that makes achieving female ejaculation so much easier.

PARTNERING QUESTIONS

When practicing G-spot stimulation, or any sexual play really, you should concentrate on raising awareness. Focus on and think about what you and your partner are doing, and talk about it. This doesn't mean that you have to plan things out in detail. Just learn to look inside, understand what you're wanting and feeling, and then discuss it. And never do anything to one another, even a long-term partner, without permission.

If you know where you and your partner both stand on sexual issues, it's much easier to relax. If you trust that your partner will respect your needs and limits, you don't have to maintain tight control all the time. Tantric Sex practitioners often focus on preparations beforehand so that we haven't a care in the world during the experience and can become thoroughly spontaneous and in-the-moment when it counts.

Trying out new things like G-spot massage and female ejaculation can be frightening or uncomfortable at first. That's why you need to practice your sexual play as a partnership involving mutual consent and equal participation as both giver and receiver. Always start a new sexual experience by discussing three issues:

1 **DESIRES:** what you want, intend, or hope will happen,

2 **CONCERNS:** what's on your mind or what you're worried about

3 **BOUNDARIES:** lines you don't want your partner to cross.

We call these the Partnering Questions.

For example, before a sensual massage a woman might ask for...

♣ long, slow, oiled strokes (desires),

♣ without things turning too sexual because she's having menstrual cramps (concerns)

♣ and with no penetration (boundaries).

PRACTICE: PARTNERING QUESTIONS

PURPOSE

The following practice guides you in getting familiar with the three Partnering Questions by discussing the topic of sex in general. During later practices, you'll use them to prepare more specifically.

1. LOOK INSIDE

Take a moment to look within and identify how satisfied you are with your current sex life. Consider what you've had, what you've got, how it's working, how it's not, plus what you want more of and less of. Include desires, feelings, concerns, frustrations, and fantasies. The more honestly you can do this, the better your coming experiences will be.

2. ONE PARTNER PRESENTS

One explains their desires, concerns, and boundaries regarding sex with the other. The other partner should simply listen, acknowledge, and ask for clarification only if necessary to understand. A minute each is usually sufficient for each question.

3. OTHER PARTNER PRESENTS

Exchange roles so the other partner can explain their answers to the three questions.

4. NEGOTIATE

If there are differences in desires or boundaries that conflict, discuss what you can do to honor each other's wishes.

PRACTICE: HOW TO TOUCH ME

This practice facilitates letting your lover know in advance what you want, where you want it, and how you want it. At last, you can reveal your innermost sensual, sexual, and erotic desires. The purpose of this practice is to let your beloved know in explicit detail how you like to be approached, spoken to, touched, and excited.

1. DECIDE

Decide who will go first. You can also decide if you both want to be nude. The first speaker can disrobe seductively if that's fun for both of you. This makes your connection playful and serious at the same time.

2. DESCRIBE AND DEMONSTRATE

Describe and demonstrate the ways you like to be approached: verbally or non-verbally, ritually or playfully, softly or roughly, or all of the above. Specifically, what kind of touching do you like where? Touch yourself in each place as you talk about it. Do you want talking or kissing or other things first? Stroke your body as you want your lover to stroke you. Demonstrate on yourself what turns you on most. You can also do the same to your partner if that helps. If you're not careful, this will probably turn both of you on. (Just kidding—no need to be careful about getting turned on. If it happens, let it!)

3. APPROACHING THE GOODIES

Explain how much warm-up your body needs before you like intense focus between your legs. What do you prefer to happen and how extensively before your genitals are approached? Do you want your butt played with, your feet or back rubbed? Don't hold anything back, whatever your preference. The clearer you are, the more likely you will get exactly what you want.

4. SHOWING OFF

Show your vagina or penis to your lover. Don't be shy! Expose all of your parts, sharing your feelings about them. Demonstrate and describe how this part of your body likes to be approached with eyes, fingers, lips, etc. Women, show your lover how to touch your outer lips, inner lips, opening, pee hole, and the inside of your vagina. If you already know where your G-spot is and what kind of stroking you like there, show him that as well. If not, it will soon be time to experiment in an upcoming chapter.

5. NEVER ASSUME

If you're in a long-term relationship, please don't assume your beloved knows everything about your body—or anything for that matter. We bet there are things you don't know yet yourself. The observer in this practice will surely learn something new, and you will too. Both of you should feel free to ask questions if something important is surprising or left out. Ask for more detail or clarification any time you're confused. While one of you is fully exposed, the other should really take everything in. You both want the new information to stick with you.

6. SWITCH

Exchange roles so you both get a chance to reveal your innermost sexual desires and preferences. By the time you have both completed this practice, you'll probably both be very turned on. Play, go for it, do what comes naturally. We never want you to miss an opportunity for a hot time together. After all, you can continue reading and learning later.

LOVEPLAY FEEDBACK

There are ways to talk to your partner that can improve your loveplay, and you've no doubt discovered that there are some approaches you want to avoid. When you think about it, the exercises in this book are a perfect opportunity to play, practice, and communicate without judgment. Let's take a look at how to make this work best.

When you're in the throes of lovemaking that's not feeling as great as you'd like, you've probably already bypassed many opportunities for sexual communication. We don't recommend calling a sudden halt to your play if you can avoid it. No matter how gently and diplomatically you confront it, interrupting pleasure can shock, sadden, and put down your lover—especially if he's male and has an ego. (And who doesn't?)

If there's something really awful your partner does once or repeatedly, talk it over when you're *not* in bed. Wait until the next day and explain how important this is to you.

Phrase your feedback around new wants and needs that you're discovering about yourself. If it seems appropriate, demonstrate exactly what you mean. This is another opportunity for the *How to Touch Me* practice!

Do your best not to indict your partner's desirability or lovability. Never compare your beloved to former lovers. Make it clear that this isn't a black mark against a man's masculinity or a woman's femininity.

So, schedule this discussion carefully. Be sure you have plenty of time to clarify and resolve the issue. If a person's ego is involved, it may take more than one session before your lover feels okay about the feedback. Keep reassuring and loving him or her throughout the process.

SEXUAL COMMUNICATION TECHNIQUES

Here are several techniques we recommend to help giver and receiver stay in close touch during loveplay or lovemaking.

"Responsiveness" and the "Feedback Sandwich" are prime tools that receivers use to guide the pleasure they're getting.

"Yes/No Questions" and "Check-Ins" are for the giver to stimulate communication when needed.

1. RESPONSIVENESS

The more lovers integrate orgasmic breathing into all aspects of their loveplay, the less verbal communication is needed. Moving, belly breathing, and sounding are a language all their own that requires few, if any, words. We call a passionate lover who shows their turn-ons "responsive." The opposite would be cold or even frigid. We wonder how many lovers have been labeled frigid when they were simply too "polite" to show their intense excitement!

So, don't hold back. Show how turned on you feel. It's exciting to let it out, and it also excites your lover. Responsiveness creates a non-verbal feedback cycle that can take you both higher and higher, and sensitive lovers who plug into your visible and auditory cues can respond to what the receiver needs and wants in the moment with little need to talk.

2. FEEDBACK SANDWICH

As you're learning orgasmic breathing, connecting with a new lover, and getting to know what your partner really wants, some talking is essential. How can you make it constructive and get what you want? Criticizing or even seeming like you're critical will be counterproductive.

For example, you may want your lover to slow down at times and speed up at others. You already know not to say "wrong — too fast" and "slow down, dummy." But if your only comments direct your lover to change speed, it's easy for them to assume that nothing they're doing feels good to you.

The Feedback Sandwich is a simple three-step process a receiver can use to constructively redirect what a lover is doing while it's happening.

A **COMPLIMENT:** A positive comment about what's going on.

B **CHANGE:** A request to try something different.

C **ACKNOWLEDGMENT:** Appreciation for how it feels better.

The Feedback Sandwich balances appreciation with coaching. In this case, it would sound something like the following:

A **COMPLIMENT:** "Your touch is so exciting. That feels really great."

B **CHANGE:** "I wonder how it would feel if it was a little slower."

Then, as soon as the touch slows down...

C **ACKNOWLEDGMENT:** "Oh, yes, that's just what I mean. That feels soooo good!"

3. CHECK-INS

When you're making love, you're a team, not a mind-reader. Just as the Feedback Sandwich is the responsibility of a receiver wanting a change, it's the responsibility of the giver of pleasure to inquire from time to time about the receiver's experience. We call this Checking-In.

Any major change in speed, position, or direction is a great spot to check-in with your beloved, i.e. "May I get between your legs so I can go faster?"

Before you enter a vagina with fingers or penis, ask, "Is your vagina ready to be visited?"

If a penis starts losing hardness, ask, "Would your penis prefer something different?"

If your lover's sounds, breathing, or motions suddenly change, ask, "Did something happen?"

These questions prompt the receiver to look inside and keep you informed about what's happening. Check-ins at appropriate times increase a giver's confidence in their ability to give pleasure. They increase a receiver's confidence in getting the pleasure desired.

4. YES/NO QUESTIONS

Check-ins are a great way for givers to ask for guidance. Yet, too much communication can bring a receiver who's relishing the sensations in their body squarely into their head, which can lose the mood.

Using yes/no questions solves this dilemma. This is the perfect response for a giver who is unsure about something or needs guidance. You can simply ask a direct question that can be answered with a yes or no or a shake of the head. This requires minimal thought process by the receiver and is much less likely to interfere with pleasure.

A series of yes/no questions can provide all the guidance a giver needs:

"Faster?" "Ah-ha."

"More?" "Mmmmm."

"Slower?" "A bit."

"All right?" "Yes."

"Too much?" "No, more."

PRACTICE: SEXUAL COMMUNICATION PRACTICE

Here's a chance to try out some of the intimacy and sexuality ideas you've communicated about in the previous practices.

1. SACRED SPACE

Use whatever ritual actions and props help you make your play space sacred. Put on sexy music that turns you on. Fill the room with beautiful scents. Put your best sheets on the bed.

2. PARTNERING QUESTIONS

Review the previous techniques about communication. Choose what kinds of loveplay you'll practice this time. Discuss desires, concerns, and boundaries.

3. RESPONSIVENESS

During your first practice session, include the four cornerstones of supreme bliss as part of your warm-up process. Put extra emphasis during your love-play on showing your excitement through your belly breaths, sounds, and movement.

4. FEEDBACK SANDWICH

Next, experiment with some new loveplay while the receiver practices using the Feedback Sandwich.

5. CHECK-INS

When you're ready to move on to the next phase of practice, encourage the giver to focus on checking in whenever you agree it's appropriate.

6. YES/NO QUESTIONS

Your next target is for the giver to use yes/no questions for minimum interruption of the receiver's reverie. When you find yourself in the midst of high passion for the receiver, the giver should use yes/no questions to obtain feedback.

7. CLOSING

Spend some final intimate time with one another to show your thanks for the trust and intimacy you shared.

AFTERTHOUGHTS

Feel free to repeat each phase of this practice several times until the techniques become second nature. After each session, share how the techniques helped or hindered your experience and how you could employ them better.

TOUCHING

ECSTASY WITH THE SLIGHTEST TOUCH

Many lovers are on the lookout for greater and greater stimulation. This often takes the form of harder and faster touching, licking, or pumping. We're going to describe just the opposite — how to train your body and your nervous system to orgasm with the slightest touch.

We call it Conscious Touch, the ultimate sensual massage through skin-to-skin contact with full consciousness. This means both giver and receiver are fully awake with all senses wide open to the physical and as well subtle energies.

A giver of conscious touch is totally present and attentive to what they're doing. They fully feel every sensation they're giving. Just being super sensitive opens the energy conduits between lovers. They focus all their concentration on flowing energy from their heart, through their arm and hand, into their fingers.

Of course, this is great advice for the receiver, too. Be totally present to the feelings, sensations, and energies.

LOVING THE LARGEST SEX ORGAN

This is more an approach to awakening the largest sex organ—the skin—than it is a technique. Conscious touch uses one of the four cornerstones of supreme bliss—presence—to magnify and enhance sensation. Your entire being reaches out from your fingertip to make love to the space, skin, and tissue of your beloved.

Conscious touch is not a deep therapeutic massage. It's soft, slow, and sensuous, usually done without oil. When many of our students begin learning conscious touch, their minds are busy, their hands go too fast, and they don't feel anywhere near what they could. This is why we teach them to begin as a meditation, emptying their minds, calming their spirits, and relaxing their bodies. Only then are the giver's energy channels open enough to flow love through body contact.

A receiver of conscious touch is far from passive. They also enter a calm, relaxed state and reach out with their senses. They put all of their attention on the feelings created in their skin. They use the four cornerstones to turn the subtle sparks that jump between the giver's skin and theirs into a waterfall of sensation.

THE FIVE S'S

As you read the various practices throughout this book, we will remind you of the most important preparations before you begin your loveplay. But for convenience, we have listed all of our suggestions here, which you might want to bookmark for future reference.

1. SUPPLIES

Before you begin, you might need one or more of the following:

- ♣ Pillows
- ♣ Props
- ♣ Water-based lubricant
- ♣ Massage oil
- ♣ Sex toys
- ♣ Condoms or other latex barriers

- ♣ Tissues
- ♣ Baby wipes
- ♣ Towels or absorbent pads
- ♣ Drinking water
- ♣ Finger-food snacks
- ♣ Music and a remote control
- ♣ Anything else you think you might need

2. SHOWERING

- ♣ Take a long bath or shower to relax you, freshen your skin, and cleanse your body and energy.
- ♣ Clean and trim your nails. If your hands (giver) are rough, plan to wear latex gloves for any kind of penetration.
- ♣ Empty your bladders and bowels.
- ♣ Beautify yourself by dressing seductively, and adorning your body with loose, sensuous clothing and jewelry (even if you're alone).

3. SETTING

- ♣ Schedule ample time without a tight schedule.
- ♣ Insure privacy and quiet, free from possible distractions and interruptions. Turn off the phones, and lock the door.
- ♣ Make sure the room is well-heated.
- ♣ Beautify your room by decorating with art, wall-hangings, flowers, incense, soft lighting, and candles, etc.
- ♣ Play soft, sensuous, or erotic music.
- ♣ Arrange your bodies to be comfortable, visible, and open to loveplay.

4. STRETCHING

- ♣ Do a little bit of stretching to promote flexibility and the flow of energy.
- ♣ A nice way to connect intimately with a partner at this point is to stretch out in a spooning position with the receiver on the inside. Then, breathe together for several minutes.

5. SETTLING

- Sit quietly, meditate, gaze into each other's or your own eyes in the mirror, share expressions of love and affection, recall times and places of pure joy, or anything else that makes you feel good.

- Ritually undress each other, whispering endearments and compliments as each part of the body is revealed.

PRACTICE: CONSCIOUS TOUCH

1. PREPARATIONS

Play soft, sensual music, and light some candles. Discuss the Partnering Questions, and decide who will begin as giver. Receiver, make as much skin available for contact as you're comfortable. The more nude you are, the better.

Start with whatever it takes to get the receiver's body relaxed and the mind present. Meditate, breathe together, and just look into each other's eyes silently. Take the time to settle in.

2. TOUCH

If you're the giver, imagine that you're extending your heart energy down your arm and into your fingertips. Rub your hands together rapidly 25 times to warm and energize them. Very slowly, and we mean very slowly, begin moving your hand over the receiver's skin. At first, massage about 3/4-inch (2 cm) above the surface. The inside of the arm is a great area for starting this practice. Believe us, both of you will feel something.

3. RECEIVER BREATHES

At the same time, the receiver reinforces what the giver is doing by using the four cornerstones of supreme bliss:

Belly breaths, deep and slow.

Sound as loud as you can on the exhale.

Movement by tightening and relaxing the PC muscle and moving the pelvis.

Presence through total focus on the sensations you're experiencing.

4. CLOSER

Now it's time for the giver to approach the skin closer. Make it as close as you can without touching, except for a few hairs now and then. Continue very slowly, moving your hand down the arm, continuing to the back or neck. This will probably be more of a powerful learning if you don't start with the genitals. We already know how sensitive they are!

5. RECEIVER BREATHES

Now, the giver focuses the mind and lets the energy flow. Touch the receiver now with complete concentration. The receiver should breathe with the giver to energize you both. Slowly, with consciousness, begin stroking the rest of your beloved's body with this sacred, ecstatic, conscious touch. This is slow, soft, deliberate, and loving with no deep tissue work, no fast pumping, no maximum friction. Follow your beloved's cues to know where to go and what to do. With the subtlest of touch, see how turned on you can both become. Enjoy!

6. CLOSING

Bring your light touch to a close. Hug, hold, or lie next to each other. Talk about how the experience was for each of you.

7. SWITCH

Switch roles right away, or take a little break first for the receiver to assimilate the new sensations.

SENSUAL MASSAGE

After all this soft work, a full sensual massage is a delightful next step. Where conscious touch provides the minimum of stimulation to the receiver, sensual massage adds maximum turn-on. Certainly, you use the two-way energy exchange you just learned, but now, you add lots of variety to the foundation of conscious touch.

Sensual massage is also soft and slow, focusing on long strokes with varying pressures and textures. Don't ignore any part of the body. Though this isn't designed to be a hand-job, brushing the genitals occasionally pumps a great deal of excitement into everything else you feel.

Vary the pressure from a light tickle to somewhat firm. Check in with your partner about what feels good, but remember, desires may change in the moment.

Sensual massage is not a therapeutic process designed to work all of the muscles deeply and alleviate body tension in that way. It's not supposed to be hard unless your partner tells you that deep tissue work creates the greatest turn-on.

We encourage the use of feathers, silk cloth, soft fur, and other items that titillate your skin. Some people enjoy rubbing with terry cloth or a hairbrush to awaken the senses. Others prefer massage with talcum powder or cornstarch for that extra sensuousness. Be sure to do this before you apply any oil, as the pasty combination isn't particularly appealing.

VARIED TITILLATION

Patting, tapping, and light scratching can be wonderful adjuncts to what we usually think of as massage. We love the butterfly, which is unexpected flitting taps with your fingertips all over the body with no pattern. Two things that turn Somraj on the fastest are scratching in the middle of his back and all over his scalp. Jeffre's favorite is tapping on her sacrum. Different strokes for different folks, right? In the next section you'll get lots of new ideas from the *Kama Sutra*.

We like to start at the periphery—hands, feet, and head—and gradually move closer and closer to center. Light, random conscious touch of the genitals is a welcome addition and great teasing for bigger things to come.

After titillating the skin with different textures and motions, ask your partner if he or she wants to continue the sensual massage with oil. If the answer is yes, remember what your goal is: To further awaken the senses and help your partner feel sexual arousal all over without concentrating on the genitals.

Many couples in today's modern world own a massage table. This can create some truly delightful loveplay. The giver has access to the whole body of the receiver with minimal stress or strain, and most any massage table will support the weight of both of you if you can't resist climbing on after the massage.

PRACTICE: SENSUAL MASSAGE

1. PREPARATIONS

Play soft, sensual music, and light some candles. Get together any props you'll need, such as oil, feathers, towels, etc. Discuss the Partnering Questions. Decide who will begin as giver and receiver. Receiver, make as much skin available for contact as you're comfortable. The more nude you are, the better.

Start with whatever it takes to get the receiver's body relaxed and their mind present. Meditate, breathe together, and just look into each other's eyes silently. Settle in.

2. TOUCH

Giver, it's now time to proceed with slow, subtle, sensuous conscious touch all over the receiver's body.

3. RECEIVER BREATHES

At the same time, the receiver reinforces what the giver is doing by using the four cornerstones of supreme bliss:

Belly breaths, deep and slow.

Sound as loud as you can on the exhale.

Movement by tightening and relaxing the PC muscle while moving the pelvis.

Presence through total focus on the sensations you're experiencing.

4. RECEIVER BREATHES

Now, the giver stroke the receiver's entire body more and more sensuously. Vary your strokes, pressure, and speed. Add patting, tapping, and even vibrating. Follow your beloved's cues.

5. OIL

If the receiver chooses, warm some massage oil in your hands, and anoint their body, one section at a time. Slip and slide with long strokes for maximum turn-on. Be sure to brush by the genitals now and then.

6. CLOSING

Bring touch to a close. Hug, hold, or lie next to each other. Feel the receiver's subtle excitement and energy. Talk about how the experience was for each of you.

7. SWITCH

Switch roles right away, or take a little break for the receiver to assimilate the new sensations.

KAMA SUTRA EMBRACES

THE INDIAN LOVE GUIDE

The *Kama Sutra* details many preliminaries to sexual union under the heading of "embraces." From that 2,000-year old text on the sexual arts, we learn how the ancient Indians developed scratching, biting, kissing, and "the giving of blows" into a high art. (They weren't talking about blow jobs at this point.)

The *Kama Sutra* cautions that people of good taste don't make these embraces violent. We don't find it particularly erotic to inflict severe pain and leave marks on your beloved's body. As we said before, some lovers are so armored against sensation that they need the strongest possible stimulation to get turned on.

In contrast, our emphasis here is to learn to use this wide range of embraces subtly to increase your beloved's sensitivity. Although not every one of these strokes is going to contribute to your personal delight or even lead you to ejaculation, we want to review some of the best for you to experiment with. You never know which ones will work best for you until you try them.

KAMA SUTRA KISSING

The *Kama Sutra* turned kissing into a glorious art form. It gave instructions about the different varieties from pecking to vibrant to rubbing in different positions and life situations. Try dry and wet, hard and soft, licking and sucking, long and short, nibbling and holding. You have many more options to play with than tongue fencing and deep throating.

Both the body and lips were fair game in the *Kama Sutra*. The Indian love guide describes "the kissing game," which is alternating the giving and receiving for maximum excitement. This makes it eminently clear that kissing isn't just for the lips!

KAMA SUTRA LICKING

Licking is juicy fun. Try many of the same variations mentioned in kissing, and try them all over. Some women especially like it very sloppy wet.

Slow is the key to ecstasy through licking. Stop if you get tired, and keep going if it turns you on. You'll have your partner moaning and groaning with pleasure, and getting very wet or hard as well.

KAMA SUTRA SUCKING AND SQUEEZING

Remember how you liked getting hickeys when you were a teenager? The edge of pain can be very arousing for many. Beware, though, that you may feel very naughty!

Think also about squeezing, which is something you can do not just with your lips, but with your fingers, your hands, your arms, your legs, and your vagina.

For all its variety of kissing techniques, licking, and sucking all over the body, the *Kama Sutra* wasn't very big on oral sex with the genitals. If you are, however, by all means, experiment.

KAMA SUTRA BITING

Biting can be light, medium, strong, or anywhere in between. Biting lips can be very erotic. The *Kama Sutra* instructed lovers to bite hard enough to leave marks all around the breast in an even pattern. These souvenirs were considered a mark of true love and an esteemed practice. We don't advocate this, but whatever floats your cork!

The teeth can be used for scratching as well. Some men even like to have their penis nibbled on. And others, like Somraj, scream bloody murder if you try it. Be careful, and start very gently. Back off if your partner doesn't like it. Always let the receiver be the guide.

KAMA SUTRA SCRATCHING

The upper class Indians grew all their nails, or sometimes just one or two, extra long. They filed them to a sharp point just for giving pleasure. Be sure to try both long and short strokes with your fingernails.

PRACTICE: KAMA SUTRA EMBRACES

As we review the various Kama Sutra embraces, you'll have a chance to experiment to discover what feels good and turns both giver and receiver on the most.

1. PREPARATIONS

Play soft, sensual music, and light some candles. Get together any props you'll need: oil, feathers, towels, etc. Discuss the Partnering Questions. Decide who will begin as giver and receiver. Receiver, make as much skin available for contact as you're comfortable with. The more nude you are, the better.

2. LIP KISSING

Experiment with kissing each other's lips and mouths. Be creative. If you get a great idea, try it out, and let your partner try it on you.

3. BODY KISSING

Extend what you enjoyed on the lips to everywhere on the body. Don't leave anything out. Relax into and relish the sensations when you're receiving.

4. LICKING

Now try licking all the parts you kissed. Use the tip of the tongue, the flat part, and the sides, and try circling your tongue on the receiver's skin.

5. SUCKING AND SQUEEZING

For another trip around the world, apply suction and pressure with your lips.

6. BITING

Experiment with biting by gently applying your teeth in all manner of places on your beloved's beautiful body. At first, stop short of leaving any marks. If requested, you can gradually use more pressure, being careful not to break the skin.

7. SCRATCHING

Your hands are dying to get in on the act, we know. Using your nails, test out different strokes, long and short, hard and soft, fast and slow, to discover what the different parts of your beloved's body prefers.

8. CLOSING

Bring your play to a close. Hug, hold, or lie next to each other. Feel the receiver's subtle excitement and energy. Talk about how the experience was for each of you. What did you like giving and receiving the best and the least?

9. SWITCH

Switch roles right away, or take a little break for the receiver to assimilate the new sensations.

MORE JUICY IDEAS

Don't worry. We haven't forgotten about our goal — female ejaculation. In upcoming chapters, you'll discover many wonderful ways to touch the vagina. But after the *How to Touch Me* practice, you should have a pretty good idea of how your woman likes her vagina approached. If not, try it again, and go deeper.

Because the vagina needs to feel safe before it can relax, the vast majority of women prefer a loving, slow approach. Women open naturally when they feel loved and desired for who they are.

ORAL STIMULATION

As we've mentioned, in spite of its detailed pro-sex guidance, the *Kama Sutra* preferred warm-up embraces leading quickly to intercourse rather than lengthy oral sex sessions.

Instead, we urge you to seek out what you like, what gets your motor running, and what makes your juices start flowing. Since arousal is essential to awaken the G-spot, we encourage you to experiment freely with oral sex. The more you play with it and like it, the more uninhibited you'll find yourself.

Get creative, and extend the spirit of the *Kama Sutra* embraces to mouth, lip, and tongue embraces. Answer the questions below, and talk with your beloved about it. Then play, play, play!

EXERCISE: ORAL DISCUSSION QUESTIONS

- ♣ The way I feel about giving oral sex is...

- ♣ My vagina or penis enjoys being kissed, licked, or sucked this way...

- ♣ Here's how my clitoris enjoys being kissed, licked, sucked, or squeezed by a mouth...

Receiving oral sex can be a powerful turn-on for both men and women, so much so that it can lead to explosive orgasms that detract from building energy and G-spot play. So, use it wisely and sparingly when you choose to expand your repertoire with female ejaculation.

CHAPTER 4

YOUR SACRED LANDSCAPE

"Transformation is through the body, not away from it."

- ECKHART TOLLE FROM *THE POWER OF NOW*

LOVE YOURSELF, LOVE YOUR BODY

YOUR SECRET RECESSES

This chapter delves deeply into the secret recesses of the female body. We begin showing you how to love and accept yourself physically. We explore the vulva, the clitoris, and vagina before teaching you sure-fire ways to discover your G-spot and move on to ejaculation. There are some darn good reasons why it's controversial, mysterious, and under-appreciated.

One study shows that 85% of women in this country are dissatisfied with their bodies in some way, while only 15% of men feel that way. Neither of these figures reflect a healthy attitude or a healthy behavior pattern.

Too many of us, especially women, internalize the media-driven pressure to have the perfect body. We want you to remember that your body is a special God-given vessel. We can wax practical and point out that it's the only one you've got and how it serves you to love it and take care of it the way it is now. But pontificating may not be enough.

Are big breasts more sensitive? No, in fact the surgically enhanced ones often lose sensitivity. Do women with thin waists have longer or stronger orgasms? No way! Does your weight influence your ability to run orgasmic energy and float non-stop in an extended orgasm? Nope, not a bit. It's really about how much you love yourself!

WHAT'S SIZE GOT TO DO WITH IT?

Penis size doesn't count in terms of sexual pleasure either, not for either gender. Sure, an untrained female lover will feel fuller when penetrated by a thicker penis. But to one with strong, supple vaginal muscles, it's not a big deal. We can't tell you how many stories we've heard about how a shorter, thinner penis used properly can hit the orgasmic trigger spot much better.

We don't subscribe to the exaggerated Madison Avenue images of what's right, healthy, and desirable. Attractive bodies can assume many different shapes, sizes, and proportions, as long as they're loved and cared for. In truth, we're more driven to the conscious presence, the life force, and the sexual energy of the beings we encounter.

Your body is the temple of your soul, the physical extension of your inner being. Forget what anyone else tries to tell you, and concentrate instead on how it feels.

TREAT YOURSELF WELL

To be totally explicit, we want to support you in feeling maximum pleasure with whatever you experience in this world, which requires that you totally accept who you are mentally, emotionally, spiritually, and physically. Your body is the physical expression of who you are in this world. It is an extension of your inner spiritual self. Loving and honoring your physical temple is demonstrated in your life through what you eat, how you exercise, and how fit you maintain your body, not to mention how much pleasure you feed it regularly.

If you desire to be a world-class lover, you must have the body and the energy to sustain frequent long lovemaking sessions. If you truly love yourself, which is a high state of spiritual health, then you will treat your body with care, give it the loving attention that is necessary, and avoid abusing it.

LOVING IT IS YOUR ONLY OPTION

Think about it. All women have a G-spot, and its power is unrelated to how they look on the outside. If your G-spot is really the secret inner orgasmic trigger to untold ecstasy, why make such a big deal about the outer?

Love every inch of your temple. Cherish and care for it. Touch and caress yourself as you would a newborn's bottom. Lovingly admire your curves, nooks, and crannies. Delight in your body's especially sensitive zones and their delicious sensations. Make pursuing what feels good your religion. Give thanks for the pleasure your body brings you. Really, we mean it!

PRACTICE: HONORING YOUR BODY

Have you ever really looked at yourself without the filter of other people's right and wrong standards? Even if you have, here's your chance to love your body fully. It's one of the things we enjoy about giving therapeutic massage. It gives you the opportunity to observe, examine, and explore every inch of your body without shame, blame, or judgment. Just accept it, baby.

1. SETTING

Stand in front of mirror in a warm, well-lit room. Play some sensuous music in the background.

2. LOOK

Look at yourself full front, side to side, back over your shoulder. Just look without judgment. Turn around in all positions and angles.

4. STRIP

Slowly, consciously, and sensuously take off all your clothes. After each piece of clothing is gone, look yourself over. Do this again and again until you're completely naked.

5. LOVE YOURSELF

Smile at yourself. Admire every part of yourself, and caress it.

6. DROP EVERYTHING

You've dropped your outer shell. Now, drop the inner ones. Ask yourself how you feel as you look at yourself honestly and completely. Leave prejudices aside whether you inherited them from magazines, movies, or your mother. Notice what beliefs crop up, and move past them by looking at yourself innocently with the eyes of a child.

7. NOTICE

Focus clearly and precisely on the details. Notice what you like about your face, your torso, your chest, your hips, your legs, your butt, your vulva or penis.

8. HEALING

Lovingly touch those areas that make you most uncomfortable. Breathe into them. Start a flow of love energy from your heart to these neglected spots. Infuse them with life by sending them love. In this way, connect every part of body with your heart and soul.

9. AWAKEN

If you can't shed some of the lingering self-distaste, energize those spots with sexual energy. Connect your rejected spots with pleasure spots. Remember peak ecstatic moments you've experienced anywhere in your body, and attach those feelings to these troubled zones. If you're concerned about a sagging breast, infuse it with the best nipple sucking you can recall. If you'd like your tummy flatter, open conduits to your clitoris by stimulating both right now.

10. BATHE

For closure, we suggest you bathe. Tidy your bathroom, light incense and candles, and add soothing salts or bubbles to the water. Then slip in with the intent of washing away self-judgments and negative thoughts about body parts. As you do, say affirmations out loud like, "I cleanse this breast of all judgment and fully accept its natural beauty and essence."

AFTERTHOUGHTS

We invite you do this practice a second time with a partner. Stand in front of each other instead of the mirror. Be sure to voice all of the positives. Say out loud what you love about your body. Second, ask your partner to voice what he or she loves about your body. Your only job is to take in the gaze, the admiration, and the love. Whatever you hear, be silent. No excuses, no self-judgments, and no put-downs are allowed. Then, switch roles.

THE VULVA

WE ENCOURAGE SELF-PLEASURE

Our fingers are the perfect natural tools to uncover the mysteries of the vulva, the vagina and the G-spot. The fingers are highly sensitive with lots of nerve endings, and we're all skilled at manipulating them. Yes, we're suggesting you touch yourself. Self-pleasuring is a powerful way to discover your G-spot and how to give it maximum delight.

We urge you not to resist any kind of sexual play. It's a tragedy that self-pleasuring isn't more socially accepted. We avoid calling it masturbation because too many people have a guilt association with the word. But call it whatever you like! Just do it. It's such an ideal way to learn about your body and sexuality. You're always the closest to the action. You have the strongest vested interest in mastering your body's uniqueness. Feedback is instant. No attention is required to the challenging art of communication, and the big payoff is immediate pleasure. Excel, and you might even have an orgasm. Whoopee!

Of course, for self-pleasuring to work well, you need to listen to your body intently instead of being consumed by guilt. To welcome the life-altering power of G-spot pleasure into your life, drop all of these old inhibitions that don't serve you. The taboos are for nay–sayers.

Unfortunately, the shape of some women's bodies makes self-plea-suring the G-spot difficult or uncomfortable. Many women's fingers aren't long enough or strong enough for facile internal experimentation. Later, we'll suggest some uses of specific sex toys to facilitate self-pleasuring. But for now, let's get down to exploring and enjoying your body by yourself.

THE VAGINA'S SACRED LANDSCAPE

Because of our social conditioning, most of us don't appreciate our genitals fully and accept their unique shape, size, and aroma. If you want to experience the heights of sexual ecstasy, it's essential that you start now on a personal program of loving these sacred parts of your body.

Right now, begin exploring your vagina's sacred landscape in greater detail. What do you think of when you look at your vagina with a mirror? A rose or perhaps a lotus flower?

Each vagina is a beautiful work of art. Just as no two women's faces are alike, every vagina is different. Some lips are longer, some shorter, each with its own special flair and personality. And remember that size and shape have nothing to do with functioning, sexual or otherwise.

PRACTICE: EXPLORING SOLO

1. PREPARATIONS

A good way to start this practice is by sitting or reclining. Tidy and heat your bathroom or bedroom so that you'll be warm enough to do this practice in the nude. We recommend a full-length mirror if you can arrange it comfortably. If not, collect a hand mirror, a strong flashlight, drinking water, a drawing pad, and some pencils before you begin.

2. BATHE

Give yourself a bath to freshen your body and cleanse your energy. Light incense and candles, and add soothing salts or bubbles to the water. Then, wash yourself tenderly as if you were bathing a newborn.

3. POSITION

Arrange yourself nude in a comfortable reclining position propped on pillows in front of a full length mirror with your legs spread apart. If you can't arrange this comfortably, you can lean against your bed headboard and use a hand mirror instead. The brighter the lighting, the better, so that you can focus on the details of your vagina.

4. SACRED SPACE

Use whatever actions and props help you to make your space sacred, including sensual music or incense.

5. ADMIRATION

Focus on your vagina with love and appreciation. Look at the various parts in depth: the hair, mound, lips, clitoris, and opening.

6. DRAWING

A wonderful way to concentrate on the details of your vagina without self-putdowns or personal resistance is by drawing a picture of what you see. Your drawing skill and art quality aren't important. It's the studying of yourself that matters. After you've sketched your closed vagina, hold the lips open with one hand while you draw the parts normally hidden from outside view.

7. TURN-ON

Gently touch the inner and outer parts of your vagina. Feel how the different tissues feel to your touch. If you want to go further, caress yourself until you turn yourself on. As you get aroused, watch the changes that occur in the skin color, texture, and shape of your body, especially your breasts, nipples, and vagina. Notice your breathing, motions, and muscle tension and other changes like lubrication. Make another sketch of your vagina when you're turned on.

8. INSIDE

Put a moistened finger inside your vagina. We encourage you to taste and smell the clean natural fluids on your finger. Learn to associate these senses with pleasure by practicing and talking with yourself. You can even draw the inside of your vagina if you've ever taken a clear plastic speculum home from a gynecological exam.

9. CLOSING

Close your sacred space by doing whatever works for you to feel good about your experience.

Were you lucky enough to play doctor with your young friends while growing up? We hope you had a chance to check out the genitals on the other side of the gender line before you bought all the negativity adults dump on kids these days. If not, never fear, you can be a kid again and play with your favorite "doctor" tonight.

If you practice this enough, you'll come to a place of personal pride. You'll believe your vagina is beautiful and really feel it is a sacred gift. So, naturally you'll want to show her off to those you love and trust.

If you've never had a partner explore your genitals in the same way, here's your chance to deepen your intimacy and self-acceptance.

Some notes to the giver: Approach this practice as a sacred trust. This kind of exposure makes a woman highly vulnerable. Tell her what you plan to do before you do it. Get permission for major changes. Maintain as much eye contact as possible. Give reassurance. If you're not sure of something, ask a question. Feedback and dialogue are great as long as you don't extend that to distracting side talk. Above all, show your love and respect.

1. PREPARATIONS

Tidy and heat the place where you'll explore your vagina to ensure that you'll be warm enough to do this practice in the nude. Have props and drinking water handy.

2. BATHE

Ask your lover to give you a bath to freshen and cleanse your energy, as well as your body. Light incense and candles, and add soothing salts or bubbles to the water.

3. POSITION

Arrange yourself with a loose wrap in a comfortable reclining position with your legs spread and propped on pillows or against your bed headboard. Your partner should be seated on a pillow between your legs. Be sure the lighting is adequate for your lover to see your vagina's details. If you want to create a better atmosphere in the room with candles and indirect lighting, your partner can use a flashlight.

4. SACRED SPACE

Use whatever actions and props, including sensual music or incense that help you to make your play space sacred. Discuss the Partnering Questions before you actually begin.

5. ADMIRATION

Spread your legs wide, and uncover your vagina fully. Ask your partner to focus on your vagina with love and appreciation, looking closely and in detail at all of its parts. The most loving partners will tell you how lovely it looks.

6. OPENING

Hold your vagina's lips open so that your lover can see the parts normally hidden from outside view.

7. TURN-ON

If you want to go further, caress yourself until you turn yourself on. As you become aroused, show your lover the changes that occur in the skin color, texture, and shape of your body, especially your breasts, nipples, and vagina.

8. INSIDE

If you have a speculum and you're willing, let your lover look inside your vagina.

9 CLOSING

Talk about how the practice made you both feel, including any insecurities or shyness that came up during the process.

TOUCH THE WHOLE BODY

The more your entire body is pleasured, the closer you will come to female ejaculation. Plus, you'll have lots of fun in the process.

The 16th-century Hindu love manual, the *Ananga Ranga*, teaches that a woman's erogenous zones are the head, eyes, lips, mouth, cheeks, ears, throat, nape of the neck, breasts, nipples, belly, back, arms, hands, thighs, knees, ankles, feet, big toes, vagina, waist, buttocks, crown of the head, and the center of the forehead. With so much territory to cover, no wonder women complain they want more foreplay!

In fact, those complainers are much more likely to tell you that it's *how* you touch their skin that feels sensual. And we're not just talking about technique here. What counts is the presence, the sensitivity, and the love with which you touch. That's the essence of the conscious touch we talked about before.

EROTIC ZONES THAT CRAVE LOVE AND TOUCH

Diving right into G-spot massage or penetration is uncomfortable for most women. Physical arousal from the outside and streaming energy from the inside are wonderful preparations for entering the G-spot.

We don't mean to suggest you should leave out loving touch of the genitals. After all, women have tissue that becomes erect, too, and we're not just talking about the nipples. Here's a run-down of the parts of the vulva.

VULVA

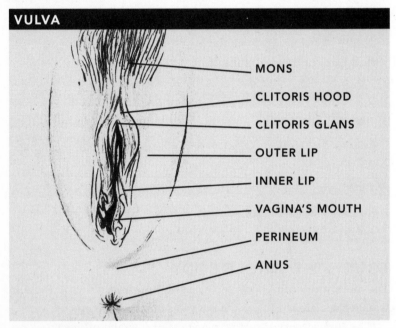

- MONS
- CLITORIS HOOD
- CLITORIS GLANS
- OUTER LIP
- INNER LIP
- VAGINA'S MOUTH
- PERINEUM
- ANUS

- ♠ **MONS:** Classically known as the mound of Venus, the mons is the soft pubic hair-adorned tissue covering the pubic bone that divides into the vagina's outer lips.

- ♠ **LIPS:** The soft folds of skin that protect the vagina when it's at rest. The outside lips are called the labia majora, and the inside ones are the labia minora.

- ♠ **CLITORIS:** The highly sensitive bud that peeks out under its hood at the apex of the inner lips and extends deeper inside around the vagina.

- **URETHRA:** The canal that conducts urine from the bladder to the outside world. You can make out the highly sensitive orifice, known as the meatus, near the top or just inside the opening of the vagina.

- **URETHRAL SPONGE:** Spongy erectile tissue that surrounds a woman's urethra composed of up to forty little paraurethral glands and ducts collectively known as the female prostate.

- **INNER VAGINA:** The elastic tube that extends from the vaginal opening up to the cervix, which is the opening to the uterus or womb.

- **PERINEUM:** The spongy, highly erogenous tissue between the vagina and the anus that includes the soft sensitive tissue on the vagina's back wall.

- **ANUS:** The other very sensitive orifice between the butt cheeks which is too often overlooked. This is unfortunate because it's loaded with nerve endings.

Just like other body parts, these erotic zones come in all shapes and sizes, which has nothing to do with their sensitivity.

PRACTICE: AWAKENING YOUR EROTIC ZONES

Let's extend your self-loving to these extra special spots. For this practice, you'll need pillows or other back support, towels, personal lubricant, a flashlight or small table lamp, and a small hand mirror. We like to put a soft towel or absorbent pad underneath to eliminate any self-consciousness caused by fluids potentially wetting the bed. Yes, your assignment, Ladies, is to get wet!

1. POSITION

Arrange yourself nude in a warm room in a comfortable reclining position propped on pillows or leaning against your bed headboard.

2. SACRED SPACE

Use whatever actions and props you need to help you make your play space sacred. Use erotic background music that gets your juices flowing and/or put flowers in the room.

3. TOUCHING

Begin touching your vaginal erotic zones slowly all over as if you've never done this before. If you can reach it, touch it.

4. EROTIC ZONES

As you glide around your skin and hair, notice what feels best, and start zooming in on what gives you the most pleasure.

5. OBSERVE

As you turn yourself on, watch the changes that occur in the skin color, texture, and shape of your body, especially your breasts, nipples, and vagina. Notice your breathing, motions, muscle tension, and other changes like lubrication.

6. MAPPING

Experiment to find what areas are the most sensitive. What kind of stroke, pressure, and speed is most erotic for each pleasure spot? What feels neutral or numb? What's uncomfortable, tense, or painful?

7. ORGASMIC BREATHING

Experiment with orgasmic breathing using the supreme bliss cornerstones to generate and spread sexual energy.

8. CLOSING

Close your sacred space doing whatever works for you to give thanks for the pleasure your body brings you.

THE VULVA-DO

Some women care for their pubic hairdo just as they do their head hair. Some tidy, some create a heart or other design over their mons, some shave completely naked down to the vaginal opening. We don't urge one form over another, but we do suggest you consider your preferences. Begin to take personal pride in the appearance of your most secret place. This isn't preparation for a sojourn at a nudist camp. It's simply about revering your most sacred of spaces for your own sense of pride.

What would look best to you? What feels best with tight pants or during sex? What does your partner prefer? Experiment and find your "pubic hair identity." We know couples who bestow the responsibility for vulva hairdos on their partner. It takes a lot of trust in your partner to allow another to take a razor or trimmer to such a delicate place.

Somraj's penis doesn't like the bristle of a growing vagina bush, both on the giving and receiving side. He trims around his penis's base every month or so to keep the wildest hairs at bay and out of the way when open access is desired. Jeffre routinely leaves just short, softer hairs on her outer lips. That's what works for us. What works best for you?

LIPS

At rest, the inner lips are normally closed like the outer lips. When a woman becomes excited, the inner lips swell, lengthen, and thicken until they protrude well past the outer lips. As a woman approaches orgasm, the lips can become red or even wine-colored.

Both sets of lips are sensitive to rubbing, brushing, blowing, and licking. Don't be deterred by any pubic hair your lover chooses to retain. Pulling on it gently and swirling it between your fingers or tongue can also be pleasurable. Just be sure to use ample lubricant so that you don't tug or abrade the skin.

WETNESS

Vaginal and G-spot massage feel much more luxurious when accompanied by ample wetness. Yet, not every woman always lubricates enough naturally for smooth gliding over all of her sensitive tissues. This is not a measurement of your sexiness or your lover's skill. It's just a physical reality like the changing of the seasons or the ebb and flow of ocean tides. Not every woman gets totally wet all the time. When a woman approaches menopause, natural wetness decreases. Plus, using latex gloves or condoms tends to dry lubrication faster than skin-on-skin play.

To learn to float in the supreme bliss of G-spot ecstasy, both giver and receiver must develop sensitivity to lubrication in each moment. Learn what brings on your natural flow and what sensual products you prefer to use for assistance.

By the way, don't hold out for the coming Female Ejaculation Chapter. The fluid expelled during female ejaculation isn't thick enough to provide enough slipperiness. When Jeffre is in a gushing mood, we have to replenish our preferred lubricant every few moments.

LUBRICANTS

What can you add to your loveplay if you need to bolster natural wetness? There are really two ways to go: oil and water. And you're right, inside the vagina, they don't mix any more than they do anywhere else.

Because they don't dry out quickly, we sometimes use massage oil or thicker oil-based products on the clitoris and the vagina's outer lips. Our favorite is actually a makeup remover found at many drugstores.

We're extra careful not to introduce any of these types of products inside. We do that by avoiding the vagina's opening at first and wiping everything carefully on a towel or baby wipe before penetration.

The environment of the vagina is a carefully balanced one, easily disturbed by introducing unnatural substances. This includes digestible items like Vaseline, oil, fruit jelly, whipped cream, chocolate sauce, honey, or even many feminine hygiene and spermicide products. One physician friend is so zealous about this that he urges women to never put anything inside the vagina that isn't pure water or their lover's skin.

Friendly bacteria, lactobacilli, like what's in yogurt, live in harmony with the vagina's wet, dark environment and keep yeast at bay. If you introduce undesirable substances, it can throw the vagina's pH balance out of whack. If the yeast takes over, the consequences are uncomfortable and sometimes painful.

The spermicide nonoxyonol, which is on many condoms and in some lubricants, is awfully strong. Some studies have shown that it's so abrasive that its use irritates the skin and makes it more likely to transmit sexually-transmitted bacteria and viruses. So, we recommend avoiding it. Further, did you know that oil-based products are known to slowly deteriorate latex? That makes them unsafe for protection against sexually-transmitted diseases when you're using condoms.

WATER WATER EVERYWHERE

There are many advantages to using water-based lubricants, as well as a few drawbacks. They tend to be more natural and more absorbent. They merge with a woman's inherent secretions better. But they tend to dry out as the water evaporates, and some have ingredients that are irritating to especially sensitive vaginas.

Though it's not as thick and long-lasting as many commercial products, saliva is the most natural, plentiful, and inexpensive lubricant around. There are lots of non-saliva choices on the market today, however. Drugstores carry a limited, often less-than-natural selection. Adult bookstores and sex shops have the best variety, but if you don't want to frequent such a store, you can buy online.

If the wetness from your vagina and mouth provides enough slipperiness for all kinds of external and internal play, then enjoy your natural lubrication. If not, or if you're curious, we encourage you to explore different kinds of substances that you can use in different situations. For instance, anal play always requires additional water-based lubrication.

PRACTICE: PARTNER AWAKENING THE VULVA

Let's take this opportunity to see what most pleases your vulva and what kind of lubrication helps. See the notes to the giver in the Play Doctor practice.

1. PREPARATIONS

Begin by tidying up, heating your room, taking a bath, and arranging the space so that you can lean back against a pile of pillows with your legs spread. Often, pillows under your knees make it more comfortable for extended play. Be sure to have drinking water and various lubricants handy for experimenting. Use soft towels or absorbent pads underneath to eliminate any self-consciousness about your fluids wetting the bed.

2. SACRED SPACE

Use whatever actions and props you need to help you make your play space sacred, including erotic music and/or incense or flowers. Discuss the Partnering Questions before you begin.

3. TOUCHING

Have your lover begin by slowly caressing, arousing, and touching you. Ask him or her to start at the perimeter and circle towards your vagina from your legs, thighs, face, neck, tummy, breasts. Make sure you both take your time and enjoy. It's your job to relax, breathe deeply, and make sounds that express what you're feeling.

4. VULVA

Ask your lover to touch your vulva with a gentle, loving touch. Giver, try circling around the perimeter and gradually coming closer and closer to the receiver's vagina. Squeeze her outer lips between your thumb and forefinger, and gently rub the outer lips together.

5. EXPERIMENT

As the vagina begins to warm and open, ask your lover to use one of your sample lubricants with different strokes. You can try oil on the outside as long as your partner is careful not to get any inside the vagina. Always ask for what you want, and give gentle, loving feedback using the Feedback Sandwich (compliment, change, acknowledge). If you don't know what you want most, ask the giver to try different strokes at different speeds and pressures.

6. STROKES

Giver, use a well-lubricated finger up and down the outside of the vagina's outer lips. You can turn this into circles by swiveling around to the other side at the top and bottom. Gradually, move your strokes and circles to the inside of her outer lips. Circle around her clitoris and her inner lips as well. Just be careful not to make direct contact with her clitoris too soon.

7. TURN-ON

If you want, after learning together, you can switch your attention to pleasure, and enjoy yourself to the fullest. Use the supreme bliss cornerstones to intensify and spread sexual energy around your body. Your partner can help by reminding you to breathe, if necessary. Though orgasm isn't necessary, if you want to end with one, go for it!

8. COOL DOWN

When you're ready to stop, be sure your partner knows to follow your lead. Do you want gradual slowing or to simply hold still? Whatever you prefer, ask your lover not to abruptly break contact. Instead, have him or her cup and hold your vagina with the palm of one hand, while the other hand is on your heart. Look in each other's eyes, and breathe together.

9. CLOSING

Close your sacred space by talking about what happened, how it felt, and by giving thanks for the trust and intimacy you shared and the pleasure your body brings you.

THE CLITORIS
THE CROWN OF FEMININE ANATOMY

The clitoris is an extensive band of highly excitable tissue whose head peeks out of the upper end of a woman's vulva just below the meeting of the inner lips. Many consider the clitoris to be the crown jewel of female anatomy. It's unique because, unlike every other part of the body, it has no other purpose but pleasure. The good news is that this spongy tissue is rich in blood vessels and nerve endings that makes it swell with arousal and become erect almost like a little penis.

The clitoris varies considerably in size from woman to woman, just as penis length and girth vary for men. The tip of the clitoris, called the glans, is located at the top of the inner vaginal lips. The glans is the part that's most sensitive to touch and averages about the size of a pencil eraser.

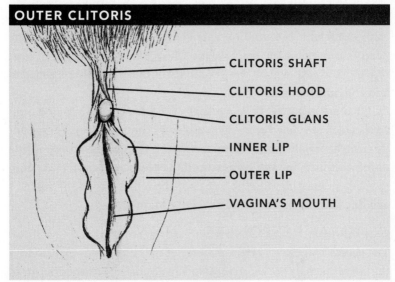

OUTER CLITORIS

CLITORIS SHAFT

CLITORIS HOOD

CLITORIS GLANS

INNER LIP

OUTER LIP

VAGINA'S MOUTH

THE HOOD OF THE CLITORIS

The intersection of the inner lips creates a hood that covers the glans and protects the clitoris. Why? Because it's the most sensitive erogenous zone in the female body. It has the highest concentration of nerve endings—as many as 8,000 in that tiny little glans. That's why the clitoris is so hypersensitive. Before sufficient arousal, direct contact with the head of the clitoris is too much and can even be painful for many women.

If you pull back the hood of the clitoris, you may or may not see it. Some just aren't visible until they swell with enough excitement. An erect clitoris often causes the hood to smooth out. When aroused, the clitoris of some women doubles in size.

When a woman nears orgasm, the clitoris typically retracts inward and downward toward the vagina's opening, hiding under the hood. But don't worry. It will reappear when arousal decreases.

THE DEEP RECESSES OF THE CLITORIS

The clitoris also has a shaft under the skin that extends up towards the pubic bone and belly before it turns down toward the vagina. When the clitoris is aroused and swollen, the shaft becomes rigid and sinks deeper inside the body.

The downward extensions of the shaft spread further towards the vagina. Some believe the erectile tissue of the clitoris extends deeper, connecting with the urethral sponge, the labia, and the perineum, nearly surrounding the inner vagina. Though this premise hasn't been proven, it would explain the sensitivity of these erogenous zones in and around the vagina.

What has definitely been medically accepted are the legs of the clitoris, which are called crura. The two crura continue deeper for about three inches (eight centimeters) toward the G-spot, one on either side of the vagina. Have you ever noticed the pleasurable sensation from two fingers pressing into the soft tissue on either side of the vagina's opening? This is one of Jeffre's favorite warm-ups.

CLITORAL RESPONSES

The deeper extensions of the anatomy of the clitoris may explain why the belief that only the clitoris causes female orgasm has endured for so long. Penis penetration may very well stimulate the legs of the clitoris. If the man moves upwards during missionary position intercourse or grinds the woman's pubic bone at the end of the in-stroke, the clitoris can receive significant excitement.

The physiology of the clitoris can help lovers understand some of the unique aspects of female sexual response. The tip of the clitoris is fed by the pudendal nerve, as are the vagina's lips and opening, the perineum (the tissue between the vagina and the anus), and the anus itself. (By the way, "pudenda" is a fancy out-of-date term for external human genitals.)

The shaft and legs of the clitoris (as well as the inner vagina and the G-spot) are fed by the pelvic nerve deeper inside. This possibly explains why orgasms feel different when triggered by the inner and outer erogenous zones. We'll talk about this much more in a subsequent chapter.

By the way, when we refer to the clitoris, we usually mean the glans. If we mean any of its inner parts, we'll be specific.

HOW TO STIMULATE THE CLITORIS

Because the clitoris is hypersensitive, begin by awakening the rest of her body. As she becomes aroused, and you approach the vagina, be careful not to directly touch the glans initially. Use a light, slow, gentle caress at first on the sides of the clitoris and the shaft. A smooth limp finger or tongue works great. Circling around the clitoris feels great, too. Be sure you have ample lubrication from the vagina, your mouth, or a commercial product. If you have really rough hands, you might like to try latex gloves. It makes the fingers incredibly smooth.

As her excitement grows, you can gradually approach the clitoris more directly. Lightly at first, your straight or circular strokes can stray toward the glans. As feedback tells you she's getting more turned-on, increase your speed or pressure little by little, and ask for feedback.

As her excitement builds, many women like a hand rubbing over the clitoris. Some like flicking with a finger or tongue. If you're using your mouth, you can try sucking an erect clitoris as well.

When highly aroused, many women like strong clitoral stimulation that's hard, fast, and with deep pressure. But be sure to ask before doing something like that.

THE CLITORIS DURING INTERCOURSE

We've found that too many women simply don't know what kinds of loveplay they like and don't like. And those who do know are often too inhibited to talk about it or just don't know how to describe it. No matter how much you know about the clitoris, every woman is different, so we encourage you to explore exactly what she likes.

Only about 10% of women have a clitoris that's close enough to the vaginal opening to be easily orgasmic from typical penis penetration. Unfortunately, in most cases, the clitoris is missed entirely during straight pumping.

By adjusting the angle of the stroking, the average clitoris doesn't have to be completely ignored during penetration. The in-and-out motion may pull the external vaginal tissue, which can massage the clitoris. And, of course, a hard penis can apply pleasurable pressure to the crura on either side of the vagina. Even better is a lover who knows how to grind his pubic bone on hers on the in-stroke. These are some of the ways the clitoris can participate actively and appreciate intercourse.

EXERCISE: DISCUSSION QUESTIONS

- How sensitive is your clitoris?

- How close is your clitoris to the opening of the vagina?

- What kinds of stimulation do you want more?

- What kinds of stimulation do you want less?

THE VAGINA

Even if you don't remember, at one time you were intimately connected with the vagina. We're sure you know the facts of life whether you recall the details of your birth or not. Childbirth, intercourse, menstruation — it seems the vagina was designed with the reproduction of the species as a first priority.

The vagina is a deeply folded, highly muscular, expandable canal lined with mucous membranes. From its outside opening between the inner lips, the vagina curves up toward the belly and cervix, which is the entrance to the womb or uterus.

Normally, the channel is collapsed upon itself so that there's no space between its touching walls. When aroused, the membranes that cover the vagina's insides lubricate. Then, it opens and lengthens.

The vagina's deeper two-thirds have smoother walls with fewer nerve endings than the outer third. Consequently, this inward area responds less to touch and more to pressure, like the kind produced by a firm, hot, cylinder of flesh. What an amazing design!

The outer third of the vagina, the part closest to the opening, is different in character than the inner two-thirds. Because it's dense with nerve endings, the walls of the vagina's outer third are highly responsive to touch. Of course, you already knew that, right? These tissues are covered with ridges and furrows, especially around the urethra that transports urine out of the bladder.

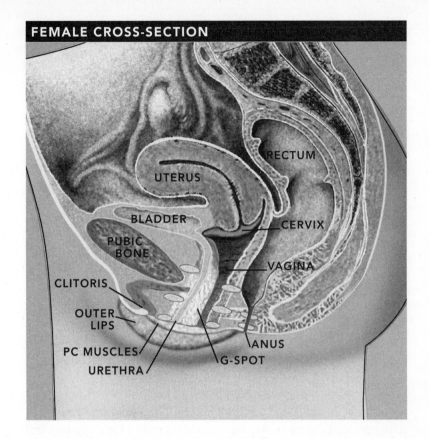

RECTUM

UTERUS

BLADDER

CERVIX

PUBIC
BONE

VAGINA

CLITORIS

OUTER
LIPS

PC MUSCLES

ANUS

G-SPOT

URETHRA

URETHRA

The bladder is above the top inward end of the vagina. The urethra is the medical name for the slender tube that runs along the top or front side of the vagina and conducts urine from the bladder to the urethral opening near the inner lips.

The average urethra is about 1.5 inches (4 centimeters) long, which is much shorter than the similar canal in a man's penis. Because it's so short, women are much more susceptible to urinary tract and bladder infections. Germs simply don't have as far to travel inside, especially after deep and extensive sexual play.

But don't worry. It's easy to prevent this. Just be sure to drink lots of water before, during, and after sex of any kind. And remember to empty your bladder as soon after sex as you can to cleanse the canal.

For many women, the opening of the urethra (meatus) is especially sensitive to stimulation since it's surrounded by the beginning of the urethral sponge.

THE URETHRAL SPONGE

There are a number of glands and tissues around the vagina that can create delicious sensations with specific kinds of massage. The tissue along the front or upper vaginal wall is colloquially called the G-spot.

The entire urethra is surrounded by spongy tissue under the upper surface of the vagina which is called the *urethral sponge*. This tissue can become erect, and the sponge is composed of up to 40 little glands and ducts referred to as *paraurethral* since "para" means beside or near.

Dr. Milan Zaviacic, a medical professor at Comenius University in Slovakia, has been studying women's urethral sponges since the early 1980s. He has clearly demonstrated that the tissue secretes the same chemicals produced by the male prostate. Since these organs also develop from the same tissue in men and women, many sexologists now use the term *female prostate* for the glands and ducts that surround the urethra.

With sexual arousal and firm pressure, the urethral sponge swells with fluid. Though the exact physiology has yet to be completely understood, it's clear that female ejaculate comes from the urethral sponge/female prostate at least in part.

Natural vaginal lubrication emanates from another source. This thicker, slippery fluid comes from the *Bartholin glands*, two small organs located on each side of the vaginal opening.

The *perineum* is the sensitive tissue between the vagina and the anus. Many women find stimulation of this area highly pleasurable because of its rich nerve endings and its ability to become erect. Plus, it's close to another one of the most sensitive organs in the body—the anus. It could be that the back wall of the vagina is so sensitive in some women because of its proximity to the perineum and anus.

THE VAGINA

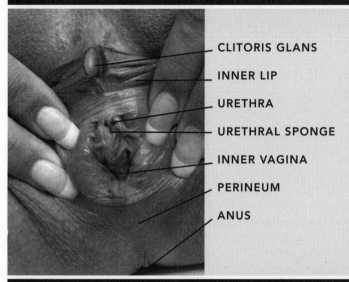

- CLITORIS GLANS
- INNER LIP
- URETHRA
- URETHRAL SPONGE
- INNER VAGINA
- PERINEUM
- ANUS

PRACTICE: SOLO VAGINA MASSAGE

This practice is a great way to discover more of the inner details you've just read about. If you have a speculum, use it. If not, we suggest you buy one. Women are undoubtedly familiar with this plastic device that gynecologists use for vaginal exams.

Reaching inside the vagina with your fingers may be awkward for extended periods of time. To prevent this from happening, we encourage you to experiment with sex toys like dildos and vibrators at this point.

1. PREPARATIONS

Begin by tidying up, heating your room, taking a bath, and leaning back against a pile of pillows with your legs spread. Often, pillows under the knees make it more comfortable for extended play. Props you may want to collect are a speculum, mirror, flashlight, lubricant, towels, vibrator, and/or dildo. Use a soft towel or absorbent pad underneath to eliminate any self-consciousness about fluids wetting the bed.

2. SACRED SPACE

Use whatever actions and props you need to help you make your play space sacred. Carefully choose soothing sensuous music.

3. BODY

Begin by slowly touching, caressing, and arousing yourself. Start at the perimeter and circle towards your vagina from your legs, thighs, face, neck, tummy, and breasts. Take your time and enjoy. Be sure to relax, breathe deeply, and make sounds that express what you're feeling.

4. VULVA

Touch your vulva gently and lovingly. As you become more aroused, add whatever lubricant you prefer. Some women prefer clitoral stimulation before vaginal penetration. Do whatever feels best to you.

5. INNER VIEWING

If you have a speculum, this is a good time to lubricate it and insert it to examine the different surfaces and glands inside. Even if you don't, you can spread your inner lips and see into the outer third of your vagina. Examine the membranes, and see if you can identify any of the different types of glands.

6. INSIDE VAGINA

Lick or lubricate a finger and slowly circle it as far as your hand will turn around your vaginal opening in both directions from 12 o'clock (the top side) to 6 o'clock (the bottom side.) Do you feel different sensations at any clock position? Does your finger feel any differences in texture or shape?

7. DEEPER

With gentle touch, insert your finger another inch, and repeat the circling motions, continuing to feel inside and out. Go deeper an inch at a time as far as you can while discovering the different feelings and sensations. Combine in and out with circling motions as you go deeper inside. Tighten your PC muscle, and feel the pressure on your finger in different positions. If your hand or finger gets too tired, remove it, and shake out the tension before continuing. Whenever you decide the time is right, feel free to switch to using a vibrator or dildo.

8. TURN-ON

To really learn what's most sensitive, switch your focus from exploring to pleasure. Use the supreme bliss cornerstones to intensify and spread orgasmic energy throughout your body. Though orgasm isn't necessary, if you get swept away by a big explosion or really want to end with one, don't hesitate.

9. CLOSING

Close your sacred space by doing whatever works for you. Give thanks for the pleasure your body brings you.

PRACTICE: PARTNER VAGINA MASSAGE

We hope you enjoyed discovering new things that please your vagina while bringing yourself exquisite pleasure. Now that you've mapped your own special zones and identified how you prefer to be massaged, you can share these findings with your partner.

Enter into this practice as a way to build intimacy rather than with any strong expectations or goals. Continue the spirit of the Play Doctor Practice earlier in this chapter.

Some notes to the giver: Approach this practice as a sacred trust. This kind of exposure makes a woman highly vulnerable. Tell her what you plan to do before you do it. Get permission for major changes. Maintain eye contact as much as possible, and give reassurance. If you're not sure of something, ask a question. Feedback and dialogue are great as long as you don't extend that to distracting side talk. Above all, show your love and respect.

1. PREPARATIONS

Begin by tidying up, heating your room, taking a bath, and leaning back against a pile of pillows with your legs spread. Often, pillows under your knees make it more comfortable for extended play. Props you may want to collect are a speculum, mirror, flashlight, lubricant, towels, vibrator, and/or dildo. Use a soft towel or absorbent pad underneath to eliminate any self-consciousness about fluids wetting the bed.

2. SACRED SPACE

Use whatever actions and props you need to help you make your play space sacred. Carefully choose soothing sensuous music. Discuss the Partnering Questions before you begin.

3. TOUCH

Have your lover begin by slowly touching, caressing, and arousing you. Ask him or her to start at the perimeter and circle toward your vagina from your legs, thighs, face, neck, tummy, and breasts. Take your time and enjoy. Be sure to relax, breathe deeply, and make sounds that express what you're feeling.

4. VULVA

Ask your lover to touch your vulva with a gentle loving touch. Giver, try circling around the perimeter and gradually coming closer and closer. Squeeze her outer lips between thumb and forefinger, and gently rub the outer lips together.

5. INNER VIEWING

If you have a speculum and you're willing, let your partner view the different surfaces and glands within the vagina. Even if you don't, you can spread your inner lips to reveal the outer third of the vagina. Ask your partner to examine the membranes and identify any of the different types of glands.

6. INSIDE VAGINA

Ask your partner to lick or lubricate a finger and slowly circle it as far as their hand will turn around the vagina's opening in both directions from 12 o'clock (the top side) to 6 o'clock (the bottom side.) Do they feel different sensations at any clock position? Does their finger feel any differences in texture or shape?

7. DEEPER

With gentle touch, ask your partner to insert a finger another inch and repeat the circling motions, continuing to feel inside and out. Guide your partner to go deeper one inch at a time as far as possible while you both discover the different feelings and sensations. Combine in and out with circling strokes while moving deeper inside. Receiver, tighten your PC muscle so that your partner can feel the pressure on the finger in different positions. If their hand or finger gets too tired, encourage them to remove it, and shake out the tension before continuing. Whenever you decide the time is right, feel free to have them switch to using a vibrator or dildo.

8. TURN-ON

If you want, you can switch your attention to pleasure and enjoy yourself to the fullest. Guide your partner to continue doing strokes that really turn you on. Use supreme bliss cornerstones to intensify and spread sexual energy throughout your body. Though orgasm isn't necessary, if you want to end with one, enjoy yourself.

9. COOL DOWN

When you're ready to stop, be sure your partner knows to follow your lead. Do you want gradual slowing or to simply hold still? Whatever you prefer, ask your lover not to abruptly break contact. Instead, have him or her cup and hold your vagina with the palm of one hand, while their other hand is on your heart. Look into each other's eyes, and breathe together.

10. CLOSING

Close your sacred space by talking about what happened and how it felt.

G-SPOT STANDS FOR GREAT

SO WHERE EXACTLY IS IT?

Just like us, we hope you've repeated the previous practices multiple times with great fun, pleasure, and learning. If you have, you've most likely discovered the supreme bliss of the G-spot, the erectile tissue inside the vagina under the lining of the belly-side wall. We call this the vagina's "front" surface since it's the inner side closest to a lover on top or in front.

But where *exactly* is the G-spot? Because it's a slang term, that's a difficult question to answer exactly. First, there are many conflicting teachings about the size of the G-spot. Some say it's the size of a pea, some say a bean, some say a silver dollar. Actually, the truth is the size depends upon the woman.

And where? Some say it's 1 to 2 inches inside the vagina or near the urethral opening. Gräfenberg, whom the spot is named after, highlighted the area near the bladder at the top end of the vagina. Others direct you midway between the cervix at the vagina's end and the pubic bone. There's some truth in all of these conflicting descriptions.

Much of the confusion and difficulty stems from the fact that this powerful "orgasmic trigger" isn't one well-defined organ like a male prostate gland or a female ovary.

Some believe the biological purpose of the spongy G-spot is to protect the fragile urinary canal from a hard thrusting penis when it gets engorged. Makes sense, huh?

TAKING AIM AT A MOVING TARGET

The G-spot is under the lining of the vagina's front wall, and it's not particularly sensitive or even noticeable without a high level of excitement. Many women report little or no feeling there at first. Some even feel initial discomfort that obviously discourages further play.

As every conscious lover knows, no two women are the same, and no one woman is the same all the time. So, unless you tune in to her unique formula in the moment, you may not feel her G-spot at all.

If all of that doesn't make it confusing enough, there are four different kinds of female prostates. In 1999, Zaviacic published his scientific findings that illustrated how the distribution of the paraurethral glands and ducts vary from woman to woman.

In most women, he discovered the greatest density of female prostate glands was located near the urethral opening. Here are the percentages of women he found with different kinds of prostates:

% of Women Location of Glands and Ducts

70% Near the urethral opening by the vaginal opening.

15% Near the bladder at the vagina's top end.

7% Midway back between the vaginal opening and cervix.

8% Minimal glands and ducts.

What this means is that your most erectile G-spot tissue is likely nearer the opening of your vagina. Even so, the deeper little "tail" of the meatus-type female prostate can be highly sensitive.

Of course, the G-spot of 30% of women follows a different pattern. There's a real chance it could be deeper inside or not very excitable without long dedicated arousal. Additionally, different parts of the urethral sponge can be aroused at different times. That makes it seem as though the G-spot is moving from time to time, even within one lovemaking session.

Visualize a clock superimposed over the opening of the vagina while a woman is lying on her back. We know the G-spot appears most often at the 12 o'clock position. But sometimes, it's found at 11 o'clock or 1 o'clock. Most sex manuals instruct us to curl a finger upward toward the vagina's front, and reach around behind the pubic bone to find the area of the urethral sponge that's particularly excitable. We now know that this doesn't contact the bulk of the G-spot for most women, although it may make its deep tail feel really good.

If you don't know which bone we're talking about, just slide your hand from your belly button down toward your genitals. (This works for men as well.) If you press inward, you'll feel the soft give of your tummy until somewhere around your pubic hair. When you feel the hard structure near the surface, that's your pubic bone. From within, you can feel the underside of this floating bone by pressing up toward your belly through the vagina's front wall.

The good news is that there *is* a surefire way to find the G-spot. Usually, the tissue covering the erect part of the sponge becomes rough and wrinkly like a cat's tongue. This is the direct result of the urethral sponge becoming engorged with blood. So, search for the corduroy, and you'll increase your chances of zooming in quickly. Couple that with searching under the vagina's lining for the little swollen glands that sometimes feel like beans, and you've got it!

Just remember not to rest on your laurels. Keep sensing with your fingertips in case it moves.

EXERCISE: G-SPOT DISCUSSION QUESTIONS

♣ How easily can you find your G-spot?

♣ What kind of female prostate do you have?

♣ What makes your G-spot swell the most?

NO LUCK WITH AN URGENT PROBLEM

As you've read, without proper stimulation, G-spot play is often unremarkable, uncomfortable, or even painful at first. Initial pressure on the G-spot can create what the medical world calls "urgency," the feeling that you need to pee. For obvious reasons, our name for this sensation is the *P-Signal*. We believe women get the P-Signal when their engorged urethral sponge presses on the neck of their bladder and urethra. Even when empty, this feels identical to the pressure caused by a full bladder.

The anatomy connection makes this clearer. Remember that the tip of the clitoris and most of the PC muscle are fed by the pudendal nerve. The bladder, uterus, and G-spot, as well as the inner part of the PC muscle, are serviced by the pelvic nerve. It makes sense that this deeper nerve pathway is harder to arouse sexually. But when it is, the sensations are felt deeper in the bladder and uterus. A woman untrained in the ways of G-spot massage and female ejaculation most likely interprets these P-Signals incorrectly.

In a later chapter, we'll explore different kinds of orgasms from different kinds of stimulation. At this point, we'll just leave you with this message: G-spot orgasms create a deeper kind of pleasure than most clitoral orgasms can ever account for.

BEGONE THAT MESSY WET SPOT!

Learning to handle the P-Signal is a vital gauntlet all women need to pass through to enjoy G-spot orgasms and female ejaculation. Now that we've launched our initial campaign to relax you about your fluid emanations, let us add a really valuable tip.

No one should have to sleep in a wet spot after sex. No one should have to hold back during sex for fear of dousing the bed, rug, or furniture by ejaculating. No one should have to avoid sex because it's that time of the month. Don't you agree? Find an absorbent towel or pad, and let yourself go.

PRACTICE: SOLO G-SPOT DISCOVERY

For reassurance, it's a good idea for a woman to empty her bladder before this kind of play. And while you're preparing, grab a couple of thick towels for that extra sense of security, just in case you ejaculate.

As we've said, getting your fingers inside the vagina with enough pressure on your G-spot may be awkward for extended periods of time. We suggest you try your best this way at first, but also have a vibrator or curved dildo available.

1. PREPARATIONS

Begin by tidying up, heating your room, taking a bath, putting on erotic music, and leaning back against a pile of pillows with your legs spread. Do this in front of a mirror if you like. Once aroused, you'll probably have to get up on your feet or knees to reach your G-spot. Props you may want to collect are water, lubricant, towels, and a vibrator or curved dildo. Be sure your bladder is empty before you begin.

2. TOUCH

Begin by slowly touching, caressing, and arousing yourself from the perimeter and circle towards your vagina. Caress your vulva and clitoris with your preferred lubricant to get them both feeling hot. Use fantasy if you'd like. Then lick or lubricate a finger, and slowly circle around the vaginal opening, gradually going deeper inside with an in-and-out stroke. Take your time, and enjoy it because your G-spot may not come out to play unless you're really turned on. Be sure to relax, breathe deeply, and make sounds that express what you're feeling.

3. LOCATE

When you're aroused enough, you'll begin to feel some places on your vagina's upper wall lining that will become rougher and more wrinkly like corduroy. You might feel the prostate harden like a bean beneath the surface somewhere between the vagina's inside end and the meatus near the opening. You won't be sure which kind of prostate you have until you thoroughly massage and excite the whole extent of your urethral sponge. Within a few minutes of continued stroking, your G-spot will swell, get larger, and harden in the same way as a clitoris and penis.

4. SQUAT

If you find you can't reach deep enough inside, or your muscles start to protest, continue on your knees or by squatting. Sometimes, experimentation is necessary to find the most comfortable position for G-spot access.

5. PRESSURE

Gradually increase the pressure on the rough and hard spots on the upper wall with in-and-out strokes about once per second. Curl your finger around the pubic bone when fully inserted, making a come-hither motion as you pull out.

6. DON'T STOP

As your G-spot becomes more engorged, you may feel P-Signals that convince you that you have to pee. This means you're really getting there! Simply breathe, and continue. If you relax into it, the sensation will pass quickly. Remember that you just emptied your bladder. If you believe it's full again, go to the toilet to make sure, but come back and resume your play.

7. TOY

Whenever you decide the time is right, feel free to switch to a vibrator or dildo. Experiment with what kind of pressure you like.

8. GO FOR IT

Use the supreme bliss cornerstones to intensify and spread sexual energy throughout your body. Of course, if you experience a G-spot orgasm, don't hesitate!

9. CLOSING

Close your sacred space by doing whatever works for you, and give thanks for the pleasure your body brings you.

THE G-SPOT DURING INTERCOURSE

We love penetration with the penis inside the vagina. But for many women, it's difficult to get good G-spot stimulation from a pumping penis. Students of the *Kama Sutra* know that certain unique sexual positions work best for different body type combinations as our later chapter will show you.

The anatomy of the G-spot is the reason. Providing enough pressure on the vagina's upper wall is necessary. This is nearly impossible with the standard missionary position. For many women's bodies, it's easier for a partner to locate and awaken the G-spot with fingers.

PRACTICE: PARTNER G-SPOT DISCOVERY

For a partner to find your G-spot with the fingers, it requires that you guide them to the right place with your preferred strokes. This is why, even if your lover knows where and how to look for your G-spot, the perennial challenges of sexual communication can get in the way.

1. PREPARATIONS

Begin by tidying up, heating your room, taking a bath, putting on erotic music, and arranging your body so that you can lean back against a pile of pillows with your legs spread. Props you may want to collect are water, lubricant, towels, and a vibrator or curved dildo. Use a soft towel or absorbent pad underneath to eliminate any self-consciousness about fluids wetting the bed. Be sure to discuss the Partnering Questions, and empty your bladder before you actually begin.

2. TOUCH

Begin by asking your lover to slowly touch, caress, and arouse your body from the perimeter and circle toward your vagina. Have your partner massage the vulva and clitoris with your preferred lubricant until they're both hot. Use fantasy if you like. When you're ready, ask your lover to lick or lubricate a finger, and slowly circle around the vaginal opening, gradually going deeper inside with an in-and-out stroke. Guide your lover to take his or her time because your G-spot may not come out to play unless you're really turned on. Be sure to relax, breathe deeply, and make sounds that express what you're feeling.

3. LOCATE

When you're aroused enough, guide your lover to explore your vagina's front wall lining, feeling for where it's rougher and wrinkly like corduroy. They might feel the prostate harden like a bean beneath the surface somewhere between the vagina's inside end and the meatus near the opening. Guide your partner to thoroughly massage and excite the area of your urethral sponge that most responded during solo play. With a few minutes of continued stroking, your G-spot will swell, get larger, and harden much like a clitoris and penis.

4. PRESSURE

Ask your lover to gradually increase the pressure on the rough and hard spots on the upper wall with in-and-out strokes about once per second. Have them curl a finger around the pubic bone when fully inserted, making a come-hither motion as they pull out.

5. DON'T STOP

As your G-spot becomes more engorged, you may feel P-Signals, convincing you that you have to pee. This means you're really getting there. Simply breathe and continue, and the feeling will pass quickly. Remember that you just emptied your bladder. If you're convinced it's full again, go to the toilet to make sure, but come back to resume your play.

6. TOY

If you liked it during solo play, feel free to ask your lover to switch to using a vibrator or dildo. If you discovered where and how you really like strong pressure, now is a good time to guide your lover to give you that kind of stimulation.

7. GO FOR IT

Use the supreme bliss cornerstones to intensify and spread sexual energy throughout your body. Allow a G-spot orgasm if it happens naturally.

8. COOL DOWN

When you're ready to stop, be sure your partner knows to follow your lead. Do you want gradual slowing or to simply hold still? Whatever you prefer, ask your lover not to abruptly break contact. Instead, have him or her cup and hold your vagina with the palm of one hand, while the other hand is on your heart. Look into each other's eyes, and breathe together.

9. CLOSING

Close your sacred space by talking about what happened, discussing your feelings, giving thanks for the pleasure you've created together.

You now know the latest information available about the nature of the G-spot, including its idiosyncrasies and its delights. You're on your way to mastering that elusive of sexual experiences—female ejaculation.

CHAPTER 5

G-SPOT MASSAGE

"Don't let another day go by without the magic touch."

— NEIL YOUNG FROM SLEEPS WITH ANGELS

TIME TO ROLL UP YOUR SLEEVES

ART AND SCIENCE

There are many ways to give ultimate pleasure to a woman's G-spot. Maybe the two of you have stumbled upon that perfect moment when his thrusts hit just the right spot. But since the G-spot's arousal is changeable, what worked once might not have worked the same way the next time. No wonder so few women have experienced ejaculation! All too often, we can't recreate the exact circumstances for that fantastic sexual high. But we can create new ones!

In this chapter, we're going to dispel the mystery about giving a woman pleasure. Here, you're going to learn the art and science of G-spot massage. We're primarily talking about using your fingers, though we'll include some guidance about using sex toys for giving pleasure to a partner as well as to yourself.

By the end, you'll know all the options. We can't promise you'll never be confused or that you'll always know exactly the perfect thing to do in every moment in every situation. As we've said, female stimulation is a moving target. But when you're done, you'll know everything there is to know about how to give and receive G-spot pleasure, and how to react to unique circumstances. It's the foundation of what you need to experience that ecstatic gush of liquid.

THE PRACTICES AHEAD

Once you've determined the pleasure formula for a specific woman in a specific lovemaking session, G-spot massage is essentially simple. There are just a lot of options to choose from in getting to that point. So, this chapter breaks down G-spot pleasure into a series of practices of increasingly complex stimulation.

You'll probably want to rush ahead to the juicier bits, and push for a resounding orgasm sooner rather than later. We understand these innate urges to seek rapid rewards. We think it's a better idea to read the whole chapter before beginning intensive practice.

Playing spontaneously, full out, with wild abandon is great. We just suggest you do it later in a few days or weeks. If you've been making love for 1, 10, or 30 years without these techniques, what's another few weeks to gradually incorporate G-spot play into your repertoire? Savor each morsel of new delight, and draw out the pleasure as long as you can.

WHEN TO START G-SPOT PLAY

How will you know when you're aroused enough for intense G-spot stimulation? The more aroused you become, the more your G-spot will become engorged with blood. It swells like a crest, protruding down from the concave front wall of the vagina, making it convex.

Until you're sure, continue with loveplay. Here's a not-so-subtle warm-up reminder: Whisper sweet everythings, kiss softly and deeply, caress everywhere, use *Kama Sutra* "embraces," and titillate the vagina endlessly. Ask your lover not to dive for the G-spot until you're really ready and ask for it.

One vital cue, however, is the vaginal engorgement. You can easily tell a vagina with erect tissues because her lips open of their own accord and become very red. For many women, lengthy clitoral play is an essential prerequisite. Some prefer touching and kissing on the vagina's lips and opening first. For some, emotional closeness, intimacy, and fantasy are enough to engorge the G-spot.

Learn your own patterns of arousal. Whatever your needs, be sure to dwell amply on awakening physical and energetic arousal before heading for the G-spot.

LEARN THE TWO ROLES

THE ROLE OF THE GIVER

As the giver, more than anything, being *present* is your most important aim. We don't just mean physically with your hands inside her. We mean mentally here and now, emotionally accessible, and spiritually conscious. Listen fully with all of your senses open. This is a powerful way to say "I love you." This is what women want more than anything else. It thoroughly turns them on.

How do you show presence? Well, tuning out, daydreaming, and looking off into the distance isn't it. Interrupting her process or disappearing in the midst of a breakthrough certainly disqualifies you.

Instead, tune in so that you notice what she's experiencing in every moment. Tell her, "I'm here for you." Respond directly to her every comment and request. And above all, maintain eye contact when she is available. She will close her eyes at times, but she needs to know you aren't checking out on her.

ALL GOOD THINGS COMES TO THOSE WHO WAIT

Another important element is *patience*. There is nowhere to go, nowhere to be, and nothing else to do but what you're doing. As we've explained, it's essential for both the receiver and the giver to drop any goals of a supreme experience or cosmic orgasm. Pushing for results can easily block them.

Just let whatever happens unfold of its own accord. Let nature take its course without fighting the current. Let sweet and gentle be your watch words.

Contrary to cultural sexual patterns or the beliefs drummed into us about what it means to be a good lover and how a "good girl" is supposed to act in bed, good sex is a joint effort. Both people need to be active partners.

Every time you connect, agree where you both want to go together using the three Partnering Questions (desires, concerns, boundaries.) Communicate what's happening in the moment. Respond to what's going on with your partner. Work together—actually, *play* together. Remember, you're the two musketeers. All for one and one for all.

As a giver, you want to reassure and comfort your partner. Be a full-time helper during G-spot experiences. When she's open to it, offer her guidance. When she thinks she knows what she wants, let her be in control. If she's struggling, assure her that she doesn't have to do it all by herself and that you're there for her.

When she's having a powerful experience, feel it with her, and enjoy it. When pleasure is your goal, not orgasm, you can only get it right and never get it wrong. Above all, encourage her to fully receive and absorb all you're giving. In the spirit of true partnership, you know you'll get yours eventually.

JUST A PILGRIM SEARCHING FOR THE PROMISED LAND

It's best if a giver of G-spot massage acts like an explorer, discovering uncharted territory. Be a pilgrim searching for hidden secrets with little in the way of maps. Stay in awe of the wonders you stumble upon.

You won't really know what she wants until it turns her on. Stay alert to her breathing, sounds, and movements. When she moves toward you and presses on your finger, she wants more. When she withdraws and pulls away, she wants less.

Be prepared for anything to happen. Your hands might be rocked violently by a bucking bronco in the throes of orgasm. You might run headlong into a hysterical outburst. You might get sprayed with female nectar. Or it may seem that nothing is happening.

You just have to accept that you can't predict the future. What worked yesterday may fall flat today. What hasn't worked for months may suddenly become the key that unlocks huge recesses of orgasmic energy. What she thought was just okay previously may be all she wants you to do from now on.

Always stay tuned for late breaking news, and you'll do fine.

ASK PERMISSION BEFORE ENTERING THE PROMISED LAND

If the G-spot is the gate to the joys of untold pleasure, the vagina is surely the garden. You don't enter such a temple without permission. You can be straightforward and say, "I'm going to put a finger inside you now, okay?" Be serious, or make it lighthearted, but don't forget: Above all else, asking before penetrating is the height of respect.

Even if you've been in relationship for a long time, ask before penetrating. If she wants to play out a fantasy sometime where you take her without asking, we think that's fine. Just recognize that she gave you permission at the beginning of your encounter. That's different than blanket permission where she gives her power away. We advise against that.

THE RECEIVER'S PREREQUISITES

At Disneyland, you need an "E" ticket for the best rides. To ride the wave of bliss when receiving G-spot massage, you need six "E" tickets. The six basic receiver prerequisites to delightful G-spot play are:

- ♣ Relaxation
- ♣ Communication
- ♣ Arousal
- ♣ Empty Bladder
- ♣ Lube
- ♣ Dropping of Expectations

LEARN TO RELAX

If you're too tense, your G-spot may not be fully open to receiving visitors. Tension can prevent you from getting sufficiently aroused to enjoy the intense stimulation of G-spot play. If you want to become more relaxed, build the tone of your PC muscle. Spend more time practicing the supreme bliss cornerstones. Do more solo exploration of your vagina inside and out. Learn to enjoy sexual pleasure through self-pleasuring.

If relaxation in sexual situations doesn't come easily to you, you might want to ask yourself where the sexual stress that blocks excitement comes from. It could be a lack of intimacy and trust with your partner. It could be that you're putting pressure on yourself to perform. Perhaps you're conflicted about sex in general as a result of conscious or unconscious social judgments and moral taboos. It could be that past abuse and wounds are creating anxiety.

In the meantime, we can only suggest that you go slowly, breathe, and allow the other receiver prerequisites to help you relax as best they can.

OPEN TWO-WAY COMMUNICATION

The more you talk about sex in general and G-spot play in particular, the more pleasure you will have — and sooner. Especially while you're learning, communicate your desires, concerns, and boundaries before you begin each session. Ask for what you want in each moment, at least to the degree that you know at this point. Give feedback supportively. If something is on your mind, let it go by talking about it. Otherwise, the inner distraction may prevent you from relaxing into pleasure.

When you're beginning G-spot play, don't worry that speaking up may interrupt the mood. Instead, use the childlike spirit of "Playing Doctor" to approach these practices in a fresh, innocent, new way. Drop any shyness, inhibitions, or judgments you have carried about sex.

As a receiver, be as responsive to loveplay as you can and use non-verbal communication to show it. The more you practice the four cornerstones of supreme bliss — breath, sound, movement, and presence — the more your partner will know what's going on with you without the need for words. You can always use the Feedback Sandwich from the loveplay chapter when you want to adjust something.

Be sure to use every opportunity to compliment your partner during your sexual antics. Since your lover will want to give you more of what you like, don't be careful about asking. At first, you probably won't recognize all of your feelings and reactions in the moment. So, it helps after each session to openly talk about what was best, what you'd like to be different, and things to try the next time.

GET HIGHLY AROUSED FIRST

As you've heard numerous times already, many lovers—both givers and receivers—have been bewildered about G-spot stimulation. Certainly, that's because it's not a fixed spot, and it often hides until awakened. Even more, we think many lovers try to push this exciting orgasmic trigger before it becomes highly aroused. We wonder how many women have found their G-spot but didn't like the sensations it produced because they weren't turned on enough.

So, embed one clear thought in your mind as you approach G-spot play, especially with a new lover: The vagina must be thoroughly and deliciously engorged first. The front wall of the vagina won't engorge without sufficient loveplay. Until this happens, any kind of touch, especially hard and fast strokes, will probably be uncomfortable, even painful, before your G-spot is fully open.

The bottom line is that you are responsible for your own pleasure. Even if you're flat on your back with your legs up, you're in the driver's seat. If you want the zenith of sexual pleasure, you have to steer. Tell your partner what feels good and what doesn't.

EMPTY YOUR BLADDER BEFOREHAND

As we've mentioned, it's important to empty your bladder before G-spot play. A full bladder makes it more difficult to relax. Not only is this sensation distracting, but there's that worry about letting go at the wrong time and making a mess. If you worry that your bladder isn't empty, you might keep your PC muscle clamped down tight. All by itself, this might stop your pleasure, your orgasm, and your delightful ejaculation.

If you're confident that your bladder is empty, and you understand that the P-Signal is normal, it will be easier for you to relax and let things go. Resting on a couple of soft towels and an absorbent pad can help free your mind of calamities, too.

USE LOTS OF LUBRICATION

We must face one of the inalienable truths of G-spot play: Dry scratching is no fun. This explains our next reminder: Get wet and stay wet.

Just like guys who tie up much of their self-image in their erections and stamina, some women connect their desirability with how much their vagina lubricates during arousal. Wouldn't it be great to always live in the fantasy of romance novels where seeing just the right bulge, hearing just the right words, or being caressed just the right way will make your vagina flow copiously?

Let's face reality. Age, health, physical condition, diet, and medication, not to mention menopause, all affect a woman's natural sexual lubrication. No big deal. Our only interest is pleasure, not giving a performance of any kind or living up to a mental image that competes with someone else.

Simply make sure you introduce lots of lubricant. Saliva is a great "wetifier." That's one of the reasons why we encourage oral romping for the longest time before G-spot play.

If oral play isn't your cup of tea, or saliva doesn't last long enough, never fear. There are many commercial varieties of personal lubricants available. Remember only to use water-based lubricants inside the vagina. Try small samples to see what you prefer.

Who's in charge of making sure you're wet enough? You both are! But as a receiver, you'll probably know that you need more first. Ask for more, or keep a bottle near you.

DROPPING OF EXPECTATIONS

G-spot play is a doorway to an exalted universe of pleasure, ecstasy, and altered consciousness. Those aren't measurable, programmable qualities. If you enter any kind of loveplay with orgasm or ejaculation as the goal, you can well block the flow of energy that will propel you higher. Ecstasy happens in the moment. Expectations take you out of it and into the future.

Yes, our goal with this book is to lead you to ejaculation, but you can't get there by trying too hard. You have to be willing to go on the journey.

The most common goal lovers set is orgasm. This can put performance pressure on you, as well as the giver. If you're worried about whether or not you will reach orgasm, you can produce performance anxiety. Trying to reproduce the excitement of a previous encounter can also distract you.

Instead, learn to enjoy the pleasure you're experiencing right now. Learn to bask in your vibrations and those of your partner. Appreciate the sensations coursing through you in the moment. Accept that whenever it stops, you'll be complete. Make what you're feeling now enough.

What's the ultimate prescription for opening the G-spot to supreme pleasure? Forget the past and the future. Focus on what's happening now.

EXERCISE: RECEIVER PREREQUISITES DISCUSSION QUESTIONS

- ♠ Consider or discuss the six receiver prerequisites:

    Relaxation

    Communication

    Arousal

    Empty Bladder

    Lubricants

    Dropping of Expectations

- ♠ What does each mean?

- ♠ What are your feelings, thoughts, and reactions to each?

- ♠ Do you have a problem with any of the prerequisites that might interfere with your G-spot play?

- ♠ Is there an alternative that both of you can agree upon?

G-SPOT MASSAGE POSITIONS

BODY COMFORT COMES FIRST

While there are limited ways to reach your own G-spot, there are several positions possible for partner play. Comfort is essential for both giver and receiver. Tension in the giver's body telegraphs quickly and can close down the receiver's energy channels.

We recommend that you experiment with the following positions before you get into serious G-spot play. Then, you'll know which to use, how to adjust them, and which to eliminate.

Once you get going with the partner G-spot massage, we urge you to speak up immediately if you find a leg going to sleep, a back in spasm, or a finger cramping. Even if you're on the verge of something great happening, don't allow the discomfort to continue.

There are six basic positions we've used for easy access to the G-spot. The first two can work equally well for self-pleasuring.

ON BACK WITH LEGS SPREAD

The most likely way for you to reach your own G-spot is on your back with your legs spread. Try leaning against a bed's headboard or other comfortable prop. Though you probably can't maintain it for long, the best access often comes with your legs in the air or your knees pressed up against your chest.

Take a lesson here from the *Kama Sutra*. One of the reasons you see so many pillows in *Kama Sutra* artwork is to provide the support needed for lengthy play. Prop up your back, neck, and head if needed. Put throw pillows under your knees. If watching erotic scenes has an affect on you, try to set yourself up in front of a mirror.

This woman-on-back position also allows easy vagina access and viewing for a giver sitting between the receiver's legs, especially if the giver moves up as close as possible. This is great for eye contact, too.

To make this position work for both giver and receiver, you'll need to deal with your intersecting legs. The giver can put both under, both over, or one over and one under the receiver's legs. As givers, we always lean against a prop of some sort and put pillows under the knees for continuing comfort and minimum physical stress. Bear in mind that you may be in this position for a while.

SITTING UNDERNEATH ONE OF HER LEGS

Wrist strain is a common physical problem when giving G-spot massage to a receiver on her back. While sitting between her legs and facing the vagina directly, the palm-up hand often gets cocked unnaturally towards the thumb. Sometimes, the giver can turn at an angle to compensate, but this complicates the conflux of legs.

To adjust even more, the giver can move outside the woman's legs. Have her leg rest over the giver's lap. By sitting underneath one of her legs, the giver can adjust the angle of the hand entering the vagina to be perfectly straight ahead. Again, move as close as possible to reduce long-term strain.

You can see why we suggest you practice before you really get into it.

LYING BY HER SIDE

Another variation of this position places the giver by the receiver's side, either lying or sitting. As before, the receiver is free to use pillows and props for maximum comfort. The giver reaches a hand over her hips and belly to the vagina. It can be difficult to avoid arm and hand strain in this position, so rest the heel of the hand on her pubic bone. For many women, this pressure is arousing and may even stimulate the vagina from the outside.

A great advantage of this arrangement is the closeness and intimacy it creates. It allows for kissing, eye-gazing, and much easier communication without interrupting the flow of G-spot stimulation.

SITTING BY THE BED

This variant of lying by her side is more comfortable for some. The woman lies comfortably on the edge of the bed with whatever cushions are comfortable for her. She can lie flat or lean back against the headboard.

The giver sits in a small chair, preferably without arms, next to the bed. If the giver's arms are long enough to comfortably reach the receiver's vagina for long periods of time, this position gives maximum comfort for both giver and receiver.

WOMAN UPRIGHT ON KNEES

When the woman is upright on her knees, she can lean forward and bend over to reach inside the vagina. So, this position works equally well for self-pleasuring. She has complete freedom to sway, gyrate, and dance as her spirit — and fingers — move her.

This stance works well for a giver seated in front of her, with pillows or other support. Because it allows such easy palm-up access, it's probably the best for G-spot discovery practices. Of course, the downside is the fatigue that may develop by balancing upright for too long.

WOMAN SQUATTING

If the receiver can comfortably squat long enough on her feet with knees bent, she provides the most open access to her vagina. Again, the giver sits in front of her, leaning against a couch or other support, if desired. Alternately, the woman can sit on the side of the giver's lap by resting one of her butt cheeks on one of the giver's legs. This lap variation also allows easy access to her open vagina.

WOMAN ON HANDS AND KNEES

Doggie-style lovemaking has a certain appeal to many lovers. Some prefer the woman on her hands and knees with the giver seated behind. Of course, in this position the G-spot is on the bottom of the vagina, so the giver's hand needs to be palm down. Spreading her weight on four limbs instead of two tends to be easier for a long-term pleasuring session, and this position allows the woman to move more freely than when lying down.

Variations on this theme include the woman with her head and belly on a pile of pillows and her bottom up for the same kind of rear entry. Then, she doesn't need to support herself on her hands and knees. She can also lie flat on her front, but this can make it difficult for the giver to reach the G-spot.

PRACTICE: EXPERIMENTING WITH G-SPOT MASSAGE POSITIONS

Instead of thinking about what would work best and debating at length, we recommend you try all of the possible positions for awhile, and listen to your body.

1. PREPARE

Read the previous section about finding the most comfortable position for G-spot massage. Collect pillows, cushions, towels, and any other available.

2. FIRST POSITION

The receiver should arrange herself as comfortably as possible on her back with her legs spread. Then, the giver should find a comfortable supported position with one hand palm up resting near the receiver's vagina and the other hand resting palm down lightly on her belly.

3. ADJUST

If you develop some strain, adjust your positions.

4. OTHER POSITIONS

When you've demonstrated how well the first position works for both of you, try the others one at a time. Be patient. It took us weeks to figure out what was most comfortable and effective.

5. FEEDBACK

When you've tried all of the positions, talk about what worked best for both of you in terms of vision, access, and comfort for both long and short sessions.

THE FOUR BASIC STROKES

GET YOUR FINGER ON IT

The four basic strokes of G-spot massage are:

- ♣ In-and-Out
- ♣ Holding
- ♣ Circling
- ♣ Come-Hither

When we refer to the giver's fingers, we use these terms:

- ♣ First finger is the index finger or forefinger closest to the thumb.
- ♣ Second finger is the middle finger.
- ♣ Third finger is the ring finger.
- ♣ Fourth finger is the little finger or pinkie.

All of these strokes can be done with one or more fingers. Because most women like the vagina to be penetrated gradually, it's often good to enter first with a smaller finger, such as the third or fourth finger. When she's opened up and wants deeper penetration, switch to the first or second finger.

Two fingers at a time are popular with many experienced women. Some prefer three, four, or even a whole fist. Be sure to ask first, though, if she wants more than one finger. For some women, too many fingers can be uncomfortable. When using two fingers, try both the first-second and second-third combinations to see what she prefers and what is most comfortable for the giver. In the proper position, a thumb works well at times, too.

After practicing each stroke later in this section with one and two fingers, you'll learn to vary these basic strokes by adjusting pressure and speed. Then, we'll show you how to interrupt your rhythm by tapping, vibrating, milking, and withdrawing to create different patterns with the arousing element of surprise.

Here is a description of the four basic strokes. As you're reading, practice with one and two fingers on your other hand, simulating the entrance to a vagina. Hold the other hand palm-down and make a circle by touching the tips of your thumb and first finger together.

By going through these motions while reading about the strokes, you'll create neuronal pathways in your body to make the movements stay with you and become more instinctual.

IN-AND-OUT

The in-and-out stroke is where you'll start your G-spot massage exploration. In-and-out is simply inserting and withdrawing one or more straight fingers into a wet or well-lubricated vagina. It probably needs little introduction, most resembling the familiar and sought-after repeated motion of a penis.

Remember to always make sure the receiver is warmed up and that you have asked permission and adequately lubricated your finger. At first, tease the inner lips, possibly rotating around the clock, with just one soft fingertip. Experiment with your first, second, and third fingers.

Once the vagina is completely wet and sucking your finger inside from your lengthy and elaborate introductory loveplay, slowly insert one finger joint, and withdraw it gently. Without a thought of rushing toward any destination, go deeper at a snail's pace until two joints of the finger are inside. Linger for the longest time, and then, continue as deep as you can reach.

Try slowly rotating your finger left and right as far as your arm's flexibility allows. With your palm up, feel all along the vagina's front wall with your finger. Can you feel the G-spot cresting? Run your finger along its middle, sides, and gutters. Can you feel the corduroy? Focus your strokes where it's most rough.

After a long, slow sojourn of one-finger in-and-out, you can insert a second one, replaying the same deepening progression. Try spreading two fingers apart so they slide along each side or gutter of the arched crest of the G-spot.

If the receiver can accommodate more and desires it (be sure to ask), continue with three and four fingers, and even perhaps your entire fist. Fisting a hot juicy vagina is an experience you'll never forget.

While you were reading, did you try in-and-out gently with your other hand? Later, we'll experiment with stronger pressures, faster speeds, and different cycles for some astonishing effects.

HOLDING

Holding means simply keeping your hand and fingers still while contacting the G-spot area. You can hold inside the vagina with one finger, two, or more, if space allows.

Holding can be done by pressing with your fingertips, finger pads, or the entire length of your fingers. You can also hold by curving your fingers behind the pubic bone, just like the come-hither stroke, except that you remain still against the front wall of the vagina.

Because it's the gentlest maneuver, holding is a wonderful way to help a woman relax and open to the intense flow of orgasmic energy. This is vital early in a G-spot massage experience. If your partner is tense, nervous, or uncertain, be sure to hold for 10 to 30 seconds each time you enter deeper with initial in-and-out strokes. Wait for signs of relaxation or arousal before moving on.

A very comforting variation of the holding stroke is to cup the vulva with your hand. This works best when the giver is lying by the receiver's side, resting a palm on her clitoris and mons.

Holding is essential when the energy becomes almost too extreme to tolerate, such as just after an orgasm.

Did you try the holding stroke on your other hand? If not, play with it now for a moment before continuing.

CIRCLING

Stop your in-and-out motion, and move your entire finger from side to side in a crescent-shaped motion like a windshield wiper motion. If you pull out slightly at one side and push in at the other, you'll be *circling*.

Try both clockwise and counter-clockwise directions to see if one feels better. You can circle with more than one finger for continuous contact on more sensitive tissues. Of course, the fuller the vagina gets, the harder this becomes. Another variation is to make circles with just your fingertips or finger pads. Once the G-spot is engorged, this is a great technique to increase stimulation.

Adding pressure and speed to circling can create wonderful sensations. As with all of these strokes, try them out on your own hand first.

COME-HITHER

Many women really like fingertip pressure on their swollen G-spot, especially behind the public bone. That's why so many lovers talk about the come-hither stroke. In actuality, it's a modified in-and-out stroke. Since it needs to go deep, for most givers, the come-hither stroke is easiest with the longest finger — the second.

To begin the come-hither stroke, the giver uses the second finger to slowly penetrate the receiver's vagina as far as possible with the palm facing toward the top of the vagina. At the top of the "in," curl the finger around behind the pubic bone. Keep that finger curled during the "out" so that it drags across the deepest part of the G-spot erogenous zone. That's one come-hither stroke.

As with the other strokes, add fingers when she's ready. Just imagine what a wide spectrum of awesome sensations you can create by increasing pressure, speed, and surprise starts and stops.

EXERCISE: STROKES DISCUSSION QUESTIONS

♣ What are the four basic strokes?

♣ Do you have any questions, doubts, or anxieties before actually beginning the practice of G-spot Massage?

♣ Are you ready to go for it?

PRACTICING THE FOUR BASIC STROKES

START WITH SOLO PRACTICE

A woman can try the four basic strokes alone as well. The truth is that once you master your G-spot solo, you can teach your partner what you've learned about yourself.

Another way to learn about the G-spot is by exploring another's. Yes, we know this may sound strange, but it's an option for those who feel comfortable with it. If you have enjoyed intimate sexual play with another woman or you're willing to experiment (all in the interests of scientific discovery, of course), doing the practices in this chapter with another woman will offer you much learning.

No, we're not encouraging you to become bisexual or a lesbian unless you are already. We just know that familiarity with the territory is essential to fully opening your sexual channels. We don't judge people for their conscious, pleasure-seeking choices.

So, if you have a close girlfriend who is open-minded, you could consider buying her a copy of this book. You might be surprised at your friend's willingness to play doctor with you.

PRACTICE: SOLO G-SPOT STROKES

Instead of approaching self-exploration in a clinical, detached way, we recommend you honor yourself in a sensual way. You're about to discover divine secrets hidden for too long.

You've already searched for your G-spot area. If not, do the Solo G-spot Discovery Practice first, or incorporate it into the following steps. If you can't make any position work quite right, skip to the sex toys practice that follows.

You do realize that your only aim here is to feel pleasure, right? Ejaculation isn't the goal just yet. Expecting mind-blowing fireworks every time is not your purpose. Remember, if you feel any physical strain, emotional tension, or strong resistance, only go as far as is comfortable, take a break, and relax.

1. PREPARE WITH THE FIVE S'S

Supplies, Showering, Setting, Stretching, and Settling. Arrange yourself in front of a mirror for this solo practice if you can.

2. STIMULATING

Caress your whole body sensuously, with oil if you want. Begin without focusing on the most erogenous zones.

3. IN-AND-OUT AND HOLDING

Using one finger, begin the in-and-out stroke slowly and gently, gradually going deeper. Each time you penetrate a little further, stop and hold until you're ready to continue. If you pay careful attention, you'll know to move on when you sense you're relaxed or feel stronger sensations. As your G-spot swells, explore its center, sides, gutters, and tail. Experiment with two or more fingers to see what you prefer.

4. CIRCLING

After you've reached as deeply inside your vagina as you can with in-and-out strokes and holding, begin circling. Try windshield wipers first, then circles near the opening, and then, go deeper. Experiment with small and larger circles until you can tell what's best for you.

5. COME-HITHER

Now, practice the come-hither stroke. Try different finger bends, depths, and angles. Try shallow, deep, short, and long strokes. Use one, two, or more fingers. See what feels best.

6. ENJOY

If you're getting turned on and still comfortable, continue, and enjoy yourself without agenda. We urge you not to press harder and speed up yet. Simply appreciate the long, slow sensual excitement you're creating. But if you want to go for it after enough subtle stimulation, don't hesitate. Celebrate any new highs, peaks, and orgasms you give yourself. And if you reach that pinnacle of ejaculation, you have reason to shout hurray! But keep reading because there's more to learn about how to repeat and intensify your experiences.

7. CLOSING

When you decide to end your session, relax gradually, and slow down your down. We really like the energy connection of one hand on your vulva and one hand on your heart at this point. Reflect on what you discovered and what felt best.

You may want to repeat this practice many times. If you find you can only feel pleasure up to a point, let that be okay. Come back repeatedly to self-pleasuring, and you may well discover your inhibitions and negative energies dissipating all by themselves. The next thing you know, you may surprise yourself with a gush of liquid.

ADDING SEX TOYS TO YOUR REPERTOIRE

As we've mentioned, sex toys help many women learn more easily about their G-spots. A simulated penis, a specially curved wand, or a vibrator may accelerate the awakening of this most powerful orgasmic trigger.

If you don't own an appropriate sex toy, you might worry about how to acquire one with minimal embarrassment. Here are some ideas:

- ♣ Maybe you have a friend who's sexually open who could advise you what to buy and where.

- ♣ You could visit one of the new breed of women-friendly adult stores. You can talk openly there to experienced women about your unique and private wants.

- ♣ Use the Internet. There are several stores, and you can order items discreetly.

USING SEX TOYS TO FIND AND PLAY WITH YOUR G-SPOT

When you choose a dildo, choose one that's long enough to reach your G-spot area. Some are designed with a bend to reach behind your pubic bone. Some are flexible, and you can bend them into just the right come-hither angle. Some come with vibrators as well. Bear in mind that the thickest dildos may be more difficult to angle toward your G-spot.

Today, you can find sex toys in all colors and materials. Be sure they're washable and that you give them a good scrubbing with soap before and after each use. The soft ones that simulate skin feel the most natural. Just be sure you don't get one with an absorbent surface. If you do, you'll need to use a fresh condom for each use to prevent bacteria from seeping into the material.

VIBRATOR LORE

There are some things to consider about vibrators. They come in all shapes, sizes, and strengths. There are erect penis shapes, wands, and eggs. You can choose from a wide variety of small battery-powered ones to those with a small wire to a battery pack. We prefer the kind that has a handle or flared bottom so that you're in no danger of losing them inside.

We don't recommend the big industrial-strength appliances with cords that plug into the wall. They produce more stimulation than you need. Vibrators with too strong a sensation can numb you out just when you want to feel more. It's best if you can find a variable speed battery-operated vibrator to adjust to your personal level of sensitivity and changing desire as you get more turned on.

The choice of shape and design are totally dependent upon personal preference. While vibrators for internal or external sexual stimulation can help you connect with the power of your G-spot, our primary concern is that you don't become dependent upon mechanical stimulation. Sure, it's great sometimes to relax and let electrical energy do the work, but you want to be able to share these pleasures with a partner as well.

PRACTICE: SEX TOY STROKES SELF-PLEASURING

If you had trouble experimenting with the four basic strokes with your fingers, we strongly urge you to try them with a sex toy. Even if you succeeded manually, why not go for it? Get yourself a couple of sex toys, and see what new things you can discover.

Remember, your purpose here is whatever pleasure you can experience in the moment. If you feel any physical strain, emotional tension, or strong resistance, only go as far as is comfortable, take a break, and relax.

1. PREPARE WITH THE FIVE S'S

Supplies, Showering, Setting, Stretching, and Settling.

Arrange yourself in front of a mirror for this practice if you can.

2. STIMULATING

Caress your whole body, long and sensuously, with oil if you like. Begin without focusing on the most erogenous zones. As you become more turned on, concentrate more on your breasts and other powerful external trigger spots. Continue your stimulation until you become highly aroused and wet.

3. IN-AND-OUT AND HOLDING

Using your chosen sex toy without vibration, begin using the in-and-out stroke slowly and gently, gradually going deeper. Every time you penetrate a little further, simply stop and hold, resting your hand on the new tissue with just a little pressure before you begin moving again. It's like a gentle introduction so there's no shock, no surprise, and no feeling of assault. If you pay careful attention, you'll know to move on when you sense you have relaxed, become more present and sensitive, or feel stronger pleasurable sensations. Don't hesitate to add more lubricant any time you feel any dryness or pulling. If you have several dildos, experiment with each of them, varying the speed and depth, to discover what you prefer.

4. CIRCLING

After you have reached as deeply inside your vagina as you can with in-and-out strokes and holding, begin circling. Try both clockwise and counter-clockwise, first near the opening, then more and more deeply. Experiment with small and large circles, as well as the windshield wiper stroke until you can tell what's best for you.

5. COME-HITHER

If your equipment allows, now practice with the come-hither stroke. This is where the curved shape of a special G-spot toy excels because it gives you leverage to reach around behind your pubic bone and drag all the way out. Try different entries, depths, and angles. Try shallow, deep, short, and long strokes. If you have a bendable dildo, experiment with various bends. See what you prefer.

6. ENJOY

If you're getting turned on and still comfortable, continue, and enjoy yourself without agenda. We urge you not to press harder, speed up, or include vibration just yet. Simply appreciate the long, slow sensual excitement you're creating. But if you want to go for it after enough subtle stimulation, don't hesitate. You may just surprise yourself with a gush of liquid. Celebrate any new highs, peaks, and orgasms you give yourself.

7. CLOSING

When you decide to end your session, relax gradually, and slow down your movements. We really like the energy connection of one hand on the vulva and one hand on your heart at this point. Reflect on what you discovered.

AFTERTHOUGHTS

We'll repeat what we pointed out before because it's so vital. You may want to repeat this practice several times. If you find you can only feel pleasure so far the first time, honor where you are. Come back repeatedly to self-pleasuring, and you may well discover your inhibitions dissipate all by themselves.

PARTNER G-SPOT MASSAGE

Now is the time for a partner to practice the four basic G-spot massage strokes. If the receiver relaxes and opens her senses as much as possible, you'll both learn a lot. To help you achieve this, we offer some reminders for both of you.

GIVER REMINDERS

Givers, do whatever you can to make your partner feel safe. Build intimacy and trust through a laid-back supportive attitude. Go slowly, and maintain lots of eye contact.

Be aware that women will know how good something feels, but they may not know what strokes you're performing from one moment to another. The nerve endings of the vulva and vagina can be hard to pinpoint for her, as the sensations run together. Explain what you're about to do, and tell her when you change strokes. Then, she can learn her own turn-ons. If you're not sure how something feels, ask her to answer yes or no questions. Adjust your strokes based on her guidance.

Pay special attention to the cleanliness of your hands at all times. Trim your fingernails short, and make sure they're smooth. If your hands are rough, use hand cream or latex gloves. Be sure to get the ones without talcum powder, which can irritate the vagina. You can also get latex finger cots, like the fingers of a glove, to cover sores or calluses. However, remember to use copious amounts of natural or bottled lubricant, especially with latex.

RECEIVER REMINDERS

Stay alert, open your senses, and communicate with your partner. Voice what you're feeling and what you want. If you're not sure about something, experiment. You can't get it wrong.

You'll see lots of references to deciding what you like best, but it's also fine if you like everything. What a repertoire you'll have to reach your ultimate goal of ejaculation! As you practice more and more, you'll become more aware of what's happening inside and what would lead you to the most intense sensations, including ejaculation.

If you're not sure about something, say so. Use the Feedback Sandwich if you want something changed. Be sure to use more positive feedback than corrections. You don't want your giver to get discouraged, right?

PRACTICE: PARTNER G-SPOT STROKES

If two women do this practice together, you'll have the chance to learn as both giver and receiver. After your first practice, take a short break, talk about what you experienced, and start afresh. Don't expect the same things to happen after you switch roles, whatever your gender.

1. PREPARE WITH THE FIVE S'S

Supplies, Showering, Setting, Stretching, and Settling.

Always discuss desires, concerns, and boundaries in the moment before beginning. Continue stimulation until she's wet and highly aroused. Remember, without sufficient turn-on, her G-spot may remain quiet and submerged. If it's not engorged enough, the giver may not be able to feel it.

2. STIMULATING

Caress your partner's whole body, long and sensuously, with oil if she wants. Begin without focusing on the most erogenous zones. As she heats up, concentrate more on her breasts and other powerful external trigger spots. Don't forget to ask permission before touching the vagina and clitoris. Be sure to use your communication skills to stay in touch and flow together. Then, continue stimulation until she becomes highly aroused and wet.

3. BEGIN IN-AND-OUT AND HOLDING

After asking permission to enter the vagina, use one finger to begin the in-and-out stroke slowly and gently, gradually going deeper. Each time you penetrate a little further, stop and hold until she's ready for you to continue. Check in verbally as often as needed to stay in sync. If you pay careful attention, even without words you'll know when to move on by sensing her relaxation, heightened sensitivity, or increased arousal. After asking, experiment with two or more fingers to see what she likes the best. And remember to add more of her chosen lubricant when there's any hint of friction or dryness.

4. CIRCLING

After you've reached as deeply inside the vagina as you can with in-and-out strokes and holding, begin circling. Try both clockwise and counter-clockwise, first near the opening, then more and more deeply. Experiment with small and large circles, as well as the windshield wiper stroke until you can tell what she prefers. Tell her what you're doing. She'll want to know.

5. COME-HITHER

Now, practice with the come-hither stroke. Try different finger bends, depths, and angles. Try shallow, deep, short, and long strokes. Use one, two, or more fingers. Ask her to tell you which area or stroke is most intense. Again, always let her know what you're doing.

6. ENJOY

If she's getting turned on and is still comfortable, continue pleasuring her without a goal in mind. Give more or less stimulation based on whether she moves toward you or away from you. We urge you not to press harder and speed up yet. Simply appreciate the long, slow, sensual excitement, but if you want to go for it after enough subtle stimulation, wonderful! There's nothing wrong with ejaculating or having an orgasm without ejaculation at this stage. Celebrate any new highs, peaks, and orgasms you create together.

7. COOL DOWN

When she decides to end your session, gradually slow down your movements. Place one hand on her vagina and the other hand on her heart.

8. CLOSING

Talk about what you discovered, and hug, kiss, or hold each other.

MAKE LOVE LIKE AN ARTIST, NOT AN ACCOUNTANT

The four strokes — in-and-out, holding, circling, and come-hither — form the basis of everything we know that vaginas like (except, of course, for penis stroking.) With the nearly endless variations on these basic themes, it can sometimes be a bit overwhelming to lovers new to the joys of G-spot play.

Think of it this way. You're a painter who wants to capture the feminine form on canvas. The variables you can employ for your creation are style, lighting, size, proportion, and color, just to name a few. With so many potential combinations, you can never decide analytically. Go with the flow, and let the creative process sweep you along intuitively.

In much the same way, both giver and receiver focus on the different variations of the basic strokes:

1 Pressure

2 Speed

3 Pattern

INCREASING PRESSURE AND SPEED

Don't forget that the vagina's deeper areas respond more to pressure than friction. That's why we'll now start to increase pressure with the four basic strokes. Let the receiver guide how much pressure she enjoys at each level of arousal. What's painful when she's just warming up can often feel quite light when she's fully aroused.

Many women find extremely strong pressure highly pleasurable when they're very turned on. Just think of how much force a big man with a strongly thrusting penis exerts. Some women have been known to get off on that kind of thing, haven't they?

Next, we'll play with increasing the speed of your basic strokes. As with pressure, speed up gradually. Though there's a place for sudden shocks and surprises during lovemaking, you need to explore this new territory first.

TEASING, TANTALIZING, OR GOING FOR IT

Instead of always pushing to give your partner the maximum excitement in every moment, use lots of variety to expand and extend the energy. We often rise to peak after higher peak, stopping with each rise to deeply feel the vibrations coursing through our bodies. It's not so much teasing as it is savoring, like sipping a fine wine versus gulping Gatorade after an intense workout.

In those times when we want to just go for it, our primary ground rule for lovemaking is to find something that's highly arousing and stick with the same stroke, pressure, and speed. In other words, if it ain't broke, don't fix it.

As a giver, you want to please. So, it's only natural that you want to go faster and harder when you see and hear how great she feels. But then, you've changed what was working. We believe that women often have trouble reaching orgasm because their well-meaning partners push for it just when the right trigger has been found. Instead of coming, she ends up numbing out because the stimulation becomes too fast and hard.

So, notice the moves that your partner loves, and keep doing it the same way until she asks for a change. You can always ask her for feedback.

PRACTICE: INCREASING PRESSURE AND SPEED

Here's your opportunity to play with increasing the pressure and speed of the four basic strokes. This practice assumes you will perform these steps with a partner. If you don't have one handy or prefer experimenting solo, by all means try this out yourself first.

Of course, add more of your chosen lubricant when there's any hint of friction or dryness. If at any time while you're increasing speed and pressure, she experiences burning, pain, or numbness, make a mental note of what caused the discomfort, and back off.

Our aim here is pleasure from G-spot massage and increasing awareness of the area in order to lead to ejaculation. But it may take some time and experimentation to get there.

1. PREPARE WITH THE FIVE S'S

Supplies, Showering, Setting, Stretching, and Settling.

Discuss the Partnering Questions before beginning.

2. STIMULATING

Caress your own or your partner's whole body, long and sensuously, with oil if she wants. Begin without focusing on the most erogenous zones. As she becomes turned on, concentrate more on her breasts and other powerful external trigger spots. Don't forget to ask permission before touching the vagina and clitoris. Be sure to use your communication skills to stay in touch and flow together. Then, continue stimulation until she is highly aroused and wet.

3. USE ALL FOUR BASIC STROKES

After asking permission to enter her vagina, use the one finger in-and-out stroke slowly and gently, gradually going deeper. Each time you penetrate a little further, stop and hold until she's ready for you to continue. Warn her as you transition to circling her G-spot first, followed by the come-hither stroke at the same slow speed and gentle pressure.

4. INCREASE PRESSURE

When you feel her G-spot swell more, cycle through the four basic strokes again, but this time, with a little more upward pressure. Explain before you change strokes each time, and be sure to check in verbally as often as needed to stay in sync. You can experiment with two or more fingers to see what she likes best with harder pressure.

5. INCREASE SPEED

Return to a gentler pressure with one finger, and cycle through the four basic strokes again. This time, however, stroke a little bit faster. Explain before you change strokes each time, and be sure to check in verbally as often as needed to stay in sync. You can experiment with two or more fingers to see what she likes best with a faster cadence.

6. INCREASE BOTH PRESSURE AND SPEED

Now that you've played with all of the basics, use your creativity to experiment using increased pressure and speed with the basic strokes. Always warning her first, try different combinations using one, two, or more fingers. Watch carefully to see what she likes and what she doesn't. Though a lot of talking may distract from her pleasure, remember that you're still exploring. Soon you'll have the tools to be synchronized and go for maximum turn-on.

7. COOL DOWN

When she decides to end your session, gradually slow down your movements. Place one hand on her vagina, and the other hand on her heart, if she likes it.

8. FEEDBACK

Discuss how the practice went for both of you. What did you both learn? What worked best? What did you learn to look out for? Does she have suggestions for the next time?

9. CLOSING

Hug, kiss, or hold each other to close your sacred space and time together.

ADDITIONAL VARIABLES

Besides adjusting pressure and speed, there are many more ways to vary the basic G-spot massage strokes. Variables in G-spot massage include different ways to start, change, and end the pattern of stroking you're using. We call them stopping, vibrating, tapping, milking, and withdrawing.

STOPPING

Stopping simply means to cease whatever motion you're doing and hold. It doesn't involve pulling out; it's simply halting your motions and holding steady in one place.

For example, you're sliding in-and-out with a fair pace and pressure when she suddenly starts shaking all over. Don't be alarmed. She's just having an energy orgasm. If you stop in this moment, she can simply focus on her inner sensations. You don't want to distract her from running the energy all over her body. That's the way she will learn how to have a full-body orgasm.

Stopping is helpful if you sense you've sped up too quickly, if you see her grimacing from strong pressure, or if you feel her numbing out from too much too fast. It helps her ground, absorb, and spread the energy that she's created, increasing her capacity to feel pleasure.

VIBRATING

Vibrating is moving your hand or fingers a very short distance extremely fast while staying connected with one wall of the vagina. It's an exciting stimulus for any erogenous zone because it simulates the quivering in the nervous system that occurs during and after orgasm.

You can vibrate up and down by intermittently putting and interrupting pressure on the G-spot. You can also vibrate side to side over the rough tissue. You can vibrate just one finger slightly, or you can move your whole hand and arm to vibrate the entire vagina. You can even use two or more fingers to spread the shaking sensation more widely. There are lots of variations of speed and pressure you can use for vibrating. Try them all, and see what lights her fuse at different times.

After some intense excitement, stopping, holding, and gently vibrating the G-spot is a great change of pace.

TAPPING

Tapping means lifting up off the G-spot and rapidly coming back down on the tissue again with some force. Tapping is most often done with fingertips but can also be done with the flat of your fingers. Though there's a whole spectrum of speeds and pressures for tapping, intense tapping is often very pleasurable.

MILKING

You can "milk" engorged tissue with rhythmic deep pressure. Hold your fingers in a come-hither position curled around the G-spot behind the pubic bone. Squeeze upward tightly as if you're trying to make a fist with your fingers. Then release and relax. This is even more intense when your palm is curled up over her clitoris and mons. As with other strokes, vary speed and pressure for different sensations.

WITHDRAWING

The contrast of intense stroking followed by a quick withdrawal of your fingers is very exciting for some women. Don't completely disconnect when you withdraw. Keeping one hand covering the vulva is a comforting way to stay with her energetically.

Pulling out at the onset of orgasm often precipitates female ejaculation. We believe this is because withdrawal relieves the pressure from the channel where the fluid erupts, while at the same time simulating the push-out of the vaginal muscles that accompany gushing.

PRACTICE: PRACTICE VARYING YOUR STROKES

Do we have to keep reminding you to ask permission, alert her to changes, and check in if you're not sure how you're doing? We hope not. We'll trust you on this one from now on. Since she's reading these directions along with you before you start, what you're planning to do won't be a surprise.

But to add in the element of surprise, explain to her that there are two actions that work much better without warning: stopping and withdrawing. Simply ask ahead of time if it's okay with her to throw these in unexpectedly.

1. PREPARE WITH THE FIVE S'S

Supplies, Showering, Setting, Stretching, and Settling.

Discuss the Partnering Questions—desires, concerns, boundaries.

2. STIMULATING

Caress your own or your partner's whole body, long and sensuously, with oil if she wants. Begin without focusing on the most erogenous zones. As she becomes turned on, concentrate more on her breasts and other powerful external trigger spots. Continue the stimulation until she is highly aroused and wet.

3. VARY THE FOUR BASIC STROKES

Begin as you did in the previous practice with the four basic strokes. Use in-and-out, holding, circling, and come-hither with one or more fingers at different speeds and pressures. Include everything you've practiced so far according to your developing judgment and your partner's responses.

4. PRACTICE STOPPING

When you sense she needs to take a breath or bask in a peak of sensation, stop all motion without warning her. With her okay, after a brief pause, resume what you were doing before the hiatus.

5. PRACTICE VIBRATING

Experiment with vibrating one finger, two fingers, and your whole hand with different frequencies and momentum.

6. PRACTICE TAPPING

Try tapping in different places with one fingertip—gently at first. Add more pressure and more surfaces, as she gives you feedback about what turns her on and off.

7. PRACTICE MILKING

At a point of peak excitement, grab her G-spot and milk it. Watch for her reaction and respond to her guidance about how fast, hard, and deep feels best. If she's really excited when you hit the perfect combination, don't be surprised if her waters flow.

8. PRACTICE WITHDRAWING

If you sense internal contractions or an impending wave of energy, draw your hand out suddenly. After experimenting in response to different signals you should get an idea about what pattern works best for her, if any.

9. FEEDBACK

During your standard cool down steps, discuss how the practice went for both of you. What worked best? Is there anything you want to remember to avoid?

10. CLOSING

Hug, kiss, or hold each other to close your sacred space and time together.

RAMPING-UP SCENARIO

You've learned the notes, scales, and chords of this new form of music, but your apprenticeship is now over. It's time to create beautiful music together with this new instrument you've mastered — the female G-spot. And the great thing about this instrument is when you learn how to play it right, you'll be rewarded with an explosion of nectar.

Seek to use your newfound skill and awareness to create as much pleasure as you can for as long as you can. Go for maximum pleasure. During this new stage of G-spot play, you may or may not have an orgasm in the classic sense. Continue to think of pleasure and ecstasy as your goals rather than orgasm, or even ejaculation. Trying too hard to ejaculate will only make it more difficult to achieve. So, just keep your consciousness focused on the whole rainbow, not any specific pot of gold. By using G-spot massage to generate vast amounts of orgasmic energy, you'll discover all kinds of new sensations. If you find yourself coming multiple times, so much the better!

CLIMBING THE ORGASMIC LADDER

Many women move up the orgasmic ladder in stages. They build some excitement, then relax, and enjoy it before going higher. You can tell when your partner wants to level off. Her motions, moans, and breath will slow down. She may even pull away from your finger.

If you sense this leveling, lighten your pressure, and slow down your strokes. Wait until she demonstrates that she wants more by heating up again or asking for it. This climbing/leveling pattern may repeat multiple times. Just stay alert, hang on, and enjoy the ride.

Should you as a giver intentionally tease your partner? Well, it might look that way to the outside observer. But what's really going on is helping your lover create and flow orgasmic energy without an agenda. For example, as strong inner convulsions begin to sweep through her, you recognize this and continue exactly what you're doing until she needs to relax into the powerful forces inside her.

To assist her ramping up higher and higher, we suggest you take on the role of ecstasy coach, reminding her as needed about breathing slowly, relaxing while aroused, moving erotically, and staying focused. Strong attention to the four cornerstones of supreme bliss — breath, sound, movement, and presence — will help her peak, plateau, and hover on the verge in order to reach higher and higher levels of ecstasy.

By the way, givers, we suggest you also use the four cornerstones yourself. Not only will it turn your partner on if you breathe and sound with her, but you'll find you have much greater sensitivity to her energy. It's a wonderful win-win if you feel the powerful orgasmic forces simultaneously surge through your body at the same time they surge through hers.

IT TAKES TIME TO SHIFT LIFELONG PATTERNS

The final G-spot massage practices employ all of the strokes and variations you've practiced so far. Your intent is to repeat them over and over and make them an integral part of your lovemaking. The more you practice, the better you'll get, and the closer you'll get to experiencing that gush of liquid. Think of the wonderful surprise it will be the first time it happens.

As your G-spot play becomes more freeform, it becomes increasingly vital to use the Partnering Questions before each encounter. Use what you learn during each session as a springboard for exploring new dimensions next time. Thorough feedback after cooling down each time is essential.

Then, before the next encounter, you can discuss new and continuing desires, concerns from the previous sessions, and any boundaries you want to set, at least for the start. Remember that establishing desires works best when you reach for general intentions like "I want to be able to relax more and absorb more sensation," rather than setting specific goals like "I want to ejaculate buckets and have an explosive orgasm within 15 minutes." Otherwise, you get hung up focusing on expectations for the future instead of fully experiencing the moment.

You're attempting to shift lifelong sexual momentum, so don't push for instant gratification. Celebrate progress with each little baby step.

Also, explorers sometimes take wrong turns, head up blind canyons, and find that they need to backtrack. Here's a good place to take the new age maxim to heart: Enjoy every step of the journey. The destination is always a varied landscape.

TWO VERSIONS OF THE PRACTICE

Two versions of the Maximum Pleasure practice follow. One is designed to help the giver develop heightened sensitivity to their partner's subtle energies and non-verbal signals. We call it the intuition-guided practice.

It's a major challenge for many lovers, men as well as women, to find out what they like. They simply don't know what turns them on, how to go about discovering it, or how to describe it once they figure it out. To ask for maximum pleasure in the moment can really stretch even those of us who think we know ourselves well.

During the second version, the receiver leads. The aim here is for her to guide the proceedings toward what turns her on when. This is a fantastic growth step for women who are accustomed to remaining passive and subservient. If they exercise the power to lead the entire sexual encounter, they embrace a whole new mindset.

Which version should you try first? Though we've listed the intuition one first, we really can't say. If you're not sure where to start, begin by alternating, and decide which is better for you at this point. Each time, be sure you're explicit about which version of the practice you're doing.

You're not just learning techniques. You're changing your sexual experience with every breath, every time.

PRACTICE: FOLLOWING INTUITION TO MAXIMUM PLEASURE

1. PREPARE WITH THE FIVE S'S

Supplies, Showering, Setting, Stretching, and Settling.

Discuss the Partnering Questions. Be clear about where you want this experience to move. Does the receiver want you to ask permission before trying certain things?

2. STIMULATING

Caress your own or your partner's whole body, long and sensuously, with oil if she wants. Begin without focusing on the most erogenous zones. As she becomes turned on, concentrate more on her breasts and other powerful external trigger spots. Continue the stimulation until she is highly aroused and wet.

3. USE THE FOUR BASIC STROKES AND VARIATIONS

Giver, according to the likes and dislikes of the receiver, employ in-and-out, holding, circling, and come-hither strokes, along with a variety of pressures, speeds, and fingers.

4. RISE TO HIGHER LEVELS OF PLEASURE

As your partner heats up and her G-spot swells, use the complete spectrum of moves you've learned to guide her to higher and higher plateaus of pleasure using pressure, speed, and interruptions.

5. LISTEN TO YOUR OWN INTUITION

Listen to your own inner signals about what she's feeling, what she wants, and what would feel best now. Whenever you're unsure, ask her for direction.

6. RESPOND TO HER SIGNALS

Giver, stay carefully tuned in to her breath, sounds, and movement. Breathe, move, and make sounds in rhythm with her to feel her energy in your body. If she forgets any of the four cornerstones, gently remind her by saying things like "Breathe" or "Relax." If she asks for something, certainly comply.

7. DON'T CHANGE WHAT'S WORKING

Once she has reached a high level of arousal, don't change what's working. If she wants something different, she'll ask or calm down. If that doesn't happen, when she's responding strongly to a stroke, move, or pattern, keep it going. Avoid the natural tendency to speed up with more pressure to make her come. More is not always better.

8. IF SHE ORGASMS

If she comes of her own accord, enjoy it. As she begins to calm down, hold still. She'll be extremely sensitive for a few moments afterward. If she wants to continue, mirror her movement when she starts moving, or ask her if she would like more.

9. CLOSING

Along with the sweet routine of maintaining physical contact, curling up together, and breathing in unison until your metabolisms return to normal, be sure to fully discuss both of your experiences. Make sure you decide what you want to do more of, less of, and practice more the next time.

PRACTICE: RECEIVER LEADS TO MAXIMUM PLEASURE

These directions are very similar to the previous practice with one major adjustment. Givers, don't do anything at all unless you're asked. If she asks for something, immediately comply. If you're uncertain, ask yes or no questions to decide what to do, if anything.

Contrary to earlier practice, these directions are written to the receiver.

1. PREPARE WITH THE FIVE S'S

Supplies, Showering, Setting, Stretching, Settling, and Stimulating.

Discuss the Partnering Questions. Tell your partner not to act without your specific instructions.

2. USE THE FOUR BASIC STROKES AND VARIATIONS

Guide your partner to employ in-and-out, holding, circling, and come-hither strokes, along with a variety of pressures, speeds, and fingers.

3. RISE TO HIGHER LEVELS OF PLEASURE

Using the entire range of moves you've discovered you enjoy, ask for different strokes, fingers, pressures, speeds, and interruptions according to what feels best in each moment in order to rise to higher and higher plateaus of pleasure.

4. COMMUNICATE

Communicate as much as your state of arousal allows. Use one-word sentences, sounds, and movements to guide your partner. If you get to the place where words distract you, give your partner permission to follow your breath, sounds, and movements. Just be sure you don't abdicate control with a blanket "do whatever you want." Instead, give a focus or direction to your partner with statements like, "Follow me deeper and deeper" or "Speed up as I speed up."

5. BE RESPONSIVE AND GIVE AMPLE SIGNALS

Use the four cornerstones of supreme bliss to continuously expand your pleasure and give ample cues to your partner. If you want, ask your lover to breathe, move, and make sounds in rhythm with you in order to feel your energy in their body.

6. FOLLOW YOUR OWN INTUITION

Be open to whatever happens, and let it be. Listen to your own inner signals about what you're feeling, what you want, and what would feel best now. Play, test, and experiment with whatever occurs to you.

7. DON'T CHANGE WHAT'S WORKING

When something really turns you on, see how much sensation you can absorb and appreciate. Remind your partner to avoid the natural tendency to speed up with more pressure when something produces a really strong reaction from you.

8. ORGASM

If you have an orgasm, enjoy it! Though a higher level of pleasure is your aim here, you can't get it wrong whether you have an orgasm or not. If you do have an orgasm, hold still at least for a moment after you go over the top to judge if you want to continue. You'll probably be extremely sensitive for a few moments, but continued stimulation may be something new that you want to experience. If you do, go for it! You may just be rewarded with an explosion of ejaculate.

9. CLOSING

Along with the sweet routine of maintaining physical contact, curling up together, and breathing in unison until your metabolisms return to normal, be sure to fully discuss both of your experiences. Decide what you want to explore further next time.

Givers may begin to feel like more of an artist with their beloved partner as the canvas. We encourage you to branch out into multiple variations in terms of speed and pressure, as well as stopping, vibrating, tapping, milking, and withdrawing.

We sincerely want you to sense the never-ending variety of G-spot play. As you integrate the attitudes of "pleasure in the moment" and "self-love as a reflection of the divine," we guarantee you'll never have a boring moment of sex play, ever again — whether you achieve ejaculation every time or not.

CHAPTER 6

SEXUAL HEALING

"Our sexuality is not only something that can be used for the enhancement of an intimate relation-ship, for physical pleasure or for procreation. It can also be used for personal transformation, physical and emotional healing, self-realization and spiritual growth, and as a way to learn about all of life and death."

— ANNIE SPRINKLE, PORN STAR TURNED SEX EDUCATOR

Sex is natural. Sex is healthy. Your mind, body, and soul can link together to create untold sexual ecstasy and bliss. Yet, few of us live an ecstatic life.

We all have the potential to achieve these sexual heights, but often, there are psychological blocks in the way. If you have little interest in sex, react negatively to sexual experiences, or have trouble letting go during sex, this chapter is for you. Even if you have a full sex life, you may find that you have difficulty achieving orgasm or feel little sensation when your G-spot is stimulated. If you fall into that category, this chapter is for you, too!

OUR TRUE NATURE

Inside each of us is a spontaneous, joyous, playful, childlike spirit who wants to be free to savor everything and love everyone. Your body is the vehicle of your soul, sexual pleasure is a divine gift, and ecstasy is your birthright.

We all naturally build up sexual energy, and it's healthy to regularly exercise and release it. How wonderful that something so good for you is also great fun.

Just like breathing and eating, sex is meant to be a natural part of our lives. But somewhere along the way, most of us lose that easygoing balance.

WHAT WENT WRONG

How did we lose our basic nature of playfulness and sexual ecstasy? In western culture, we're taught that our sexual energies are dangerous. We're made to believe that we must contain our sexuality and keep it in check. We're made to live unnaturally by social conditioning and moral codes that don't serve our inherent make-up. All the do's and don'ts of human society produce inner struggles against our basic desires. The next thing we know, our sexual energies are in a cage, and this contributes to the difficulties of enjoying G-spot play, orgasmic energy, and female ejaculation.

Growing up in our sexually immature and repressed society, none of us can avoid accumulating energetic sexual blocks. We're lectured to, corrected, and made wrong for our instincts and natural proclivities.

At young and vulnerable ages, we wade into the scary arena of sexuality largely unprepared and uneducated. In other words ... ignorant.

We're peppered with learning taboos, injunctions, and the multifarious definitions of the sins of the flesh. Often, it's religious imprinting that creates these huge inhibitions and enormous loads of guilt and shame.

Women and men who've been sexually exploited, abused, and wounded may carry even more baggage. This negative energy is held in the G-spot. For too many, carrying this baggage gets in the way of enjoyment, orgasm, and ejaculation.

DON'T RUN OR HIDE — PLAY!

Do you want to become sexually whole? Do you hope to experience more and more sexual pleasure? Do you look forward to higher and higher peaks of sexual ecstasy?

To fully open to the joys of sexuality requires a clearing of negative programming. We all have varying degrees of sexual negativity to clear, but trust us—it can be done!

So, how do you shed the social conventions that bring you down? How do you release the guilt that keeps you boxed in? How do you heal old wounds? Healing and letting go into the pleasures of sex are what this chapter are all about. It's the precursor to achieving ejaculation. If you have any blocks that prevent you from experiencing this "letting go" from your G-spot, the work you do as a result of this chapter will help you reach your goal and much more.

EXERCISE: OPENING DISCUSSION QUESTIONS

- What do you feel is your basic nature?

- Do you remember when you felt fully open and alive? How old were you?

- What did you learn that helped you shut down to that childlike playfulness?

SEXUAL RESISTANCE

When we relax, exercise our erogenous zones, and enjoy our bodies, we often run into the old baggage that blocks excitement and pleasure.

We've all been through one or another of these scenarios:

- You meet someone you find very attractive. You finally get to the big moment in bed, and either your energy isn't there, or your new lover's desire goes flat. What happened?

- You've been thinking about sex for days, and now, you finally have the opportunity. But suddenly, you end up in an argument, and sex and communion become the last thing either of you wants.

- You're a hot and sexy lover, and you fall for a wonderful guy or gal. You absolutely adore oral sex, but he won't taste your vagina, or she won't taste your penis. Now, what do you do?

♣ At last, you've fallen for your dream lover. The first six months are fabulous: juicy days and hotter nights. Then, for no apparent reason, she's no longer interested in sex, or his erections take a vacation.

♣ You marry even though you know your spouse doesn't have much of a sex drive. You hope it will change, or you tell yourself that it isn't important. Too often, it doesn't change, and in the long run, it really is important, isn't it?

What do all of these situations have in common? Sexual resistance has reared its ugly head.

WHAT IS RESISTANCE?

Resistance is anything that gets in the way of the natural flow of life force energy. That's why we coined the phrase "liquid mind, liquid body."

Remember a time when you felt vibrant, alive, eager, and joyful about every little thing. Your life force was certainly flowing then! When you're feeling good, which is your basic nature, energy flows continuously. Sexual pleasure, orgasm, and ejaculation are prime examples. When your energetic juices are flowing, your emotions are upbeat, your body is dynamic, your mind is clear, and your spirit soars.

When your energy is inhibited, there is resistance and blockage. Then, you feel turned off, repulsed, angry, irritated, frustrated, hopeless, or depressed. In fact, you can define your own resistance by the very times you feel these so-called negative feelings.

ISSUES IN THE TISSUES

Of course, you're aware that upsets, disappointments, and other negative emotions can come back to haunt you. Did you know that these old emotions settle in your body? Did you know that pains, wounds, and trauma are stored deep in your tissues? We often call this "body memory."

You want to feel pleasure, you want to enjoy the sunset, and you want to shower your beloved with affection, but something gets in your way. Sometimes, the very attempt to flow positive energy brings old sad stories up from your body memory and creates resistance.

That's partly why we're all so starved for touch. It's why massage and sexual dalliance feel so good. These are natural soothing mechanisms that strive to relieve the stress and tension buried in our bodies.

In short, resistance comes from energy blocked in the body that inhibits love, joy, pleasure, sexual abandon, and even orgasm and ejaculation.

WHERE DOES RESISTANCE COME FROM?

Resistance comes from internal conflict. Psychologically, it's caused by thoughts, beliefs, and feelings that are in conflict with what you want. These inner inhibitions may block you from being sexual, giving and receiving love, or making a relationship commitment. You might just feel uncomfortable about something, or you may experience some form of fear, anxiety, or even inexplicable anger. Either way, it's not a liquid mental state.

Why would you inhibit your own natural desires?

- Maybe you're feeling down about not having what you want or what you think you should have.
- Maybe you have high standards and expect more of yourself and others.
- Maybe you feel there's something wrong with what you want.
- Maybe you're pushing to achieve a goal and doubt your ability to reach it.
- Maybe you believe there's something wrong with you and that anything you might want is dirty, bad, or evil.

Resistance usually stems from deeply internalized rules about enjoying life and sex, and these rules get in the way of pleasure. Sadly, society as a whole seems to believe it's dangerous to live an ecstatic life.

BLOCKING THE SEXUAL STIMULATION PATHWAY

What's the most powerful sex organ in your body? Your guessed it—your brain.

When everything is functioning properly, energy is flowing. You have a desire borne of love, lust, an image, a touch, or a fantasy. In response, the automatic mechanisms of your body create arousal.

As you begin to experience good feelings, the autonomic nervous system carries those messages back to the pleasure centers of the brain to create a feedback loop. In other words, when you get turned on, you get more and more turned on without much effort. This works in arenas other than sex as well.

Of course, this assumes that your conscious mind doesn't interfere in any way and lets your body take over. When you welcome the desire, your energy flow creates passion.

When you have some built-in resistance, your beliefs and feelings conflict with this blessed human process of arousal. Consciously or unconsciously, you think, "Nice girls don't" or "I shouldn't" or "It's not right." The vibrations of these resistant beliefs block the natural flow of messages to and from the brain. The feedback loop is stopped in its tracks, and your excitement wanes.

If this pattern isn't modified, your pleasure channels shut down. The old maxim "use it or lose it" applies more to sexuality than other parts of life.

When you aren't really conscious of the resistance mechanism at work, these confusing mixed messages can make both giver and receiver crazy. You might feel nervous, anxious, afraid, angry, or withdrawn without any logical explanation. Your old emotional baggage leads you without your understanding what's happening.

Ever wonder why we sometimes inexplicably find ourselves laughing, crying, swooning, or screaming during sex? We've touched a nerve from some past wound.

FLOW WITH THE STREAM

To grasp the dynamics of internal resistance, picture a flowing mountain stream. In mid-summer, it runs quietly along the rocks, banks, and bottom. When the spring flood arrives, the force of the water causes deep turbulence. Rocks, logs, and the very banks themselves are battered and often swept away.

Internal resistance to energy flow is like an obstacle in the path of a stream. Doesn't it feel like you're emotionally battered and churned up by stress? Doesn't it feel like you're pushed around by conflicting tides?

When you push psychically against something in your life, your immune system can easily go out of balance, making you vulnerable to disease. Instead of liquid and flowing, your resistant mind makes your body struggle.

You can soften the brunt of resistance by choosing to mute your desire for living, ignore your senses, and avoid pleasure. Then there's less force battering the stream bed. But you'll slowly create less and less of the enjoyment that is part and parcel of your life force. We don't recommend hiding away in a cave, sticking your head in the sand, or avoiding what's bugging you.

By the way, this explains why a high stress lifestyle can inhibit your sexual desire and your sexual performance over time. The stress you feel within is just another form of resistance. For example, if you place high expectations on yourself (although it may feel like others are doing this), you may have trouble living up to your own demands.

Many of those suffering from sexual resistance distract themselves by total immersion in work, family, investments, etc. A high stress lifestyle can be just another manifestation of resistance, sucking a person dry of any energy or time they could use to experience pleasure.

SPECIFIC CAUSES OF RESISTANCE

Though you're probably all too aware of many of the resistances in your life, we've compiled a short list to broaden your understanding of the possible ways your past can get in the way of your present. Though sexual abuse and child molestation are popular news items these days, there are many other ways in which women, as well as men, collect emotional wounding and physical trauma.

FEARS

What we worry about often becomes a self-fulfilling prophecy. From embarrassing discoveries like our first underarm and pubic hairs, wet dreams, or menstruation to our first fumbling sexual encounters, our inexperience and ignorance causes us to worry about making a fool of ourselves. Without education to prepare us to love and accept who we are, our bodies and what others might think about us seems awfully scary.

SOCIAL CONDITIONING

Strict social, religious, and cultural puritanical attitudes create injunctions, prohibitions, and taboos which conflict with our healthy impulses. When we learn them from authority figures like parents, teachers, religious leaders, neighbors, and friends, they carry extra weight. We end up feeling ashamed, blamed, and accused for trying to deal with the life forces burbling inside. Even worse, victims of abuse are often not believed or made to feel wrong.

GUILT

When we accept our elders' beliefs, such as "Don't touch yourself there or you'll go to hell," we end up loaded with guilt. Who hasn't been saddled with guilt by pushing too hard for sex, saying no when we mean yes, or not knowing how to satisfy a lover and feeling inadequate? The biological imperatives of love, lust, and intimacy drive us to act, and then we regret being human.

SELF-JUDGMENT

Maybe the most damaging impact comes from judging ourselves. We explore our bodies, play doctor with friends, and discover how to give ourselves pleasure. All of these explorations are innocent, but then, we learn "it was wrong." We become disgusted with our bodies and their natural secretions. We condemn our own genitals as sinful, dirty, or base, and these unfair negative self-judgments may end up deeply repressed and outside our adult awareness.

PAINFUL INCIDENTS

When we experience physical ailments in our sensitive areas, they leave lasting imprints. The pain of parental punishments, abusive relationships, infidelities, severe losses, and other violent incidents run deep. We all dread the stories of sexual violence like rape and incest, but even common life experiences like childbirth, abortion, miscarriage, and insensitive gynecological exams can also contribute.

UNWANTED SEX

If it wasn't bad enough growing up with all of these pains, power trips, and mind games that society lays on us, who hasn't experienced some kind of harassment in our sexually distorted world? How many innocents have been mistreated, exploited, used, or violated? Who hasn't been pressured, forced, or overpowered to do something they didn't want to do?

This is just a brief survey of the many ways our sexually repressive culture has contributed to the resistance we carry around with us. But remember, the outside events, however damaging, can't produce harmful energetic scar tissue unless we store them deep within, never letting the light shine on them.

ARMORING

When past traumatic experiences are lodged in the body's muscles, they tighten, and the surrounding tissues harden. Some call this "armoring."

Armoring is an attempt to prevent pain. We tighten and contract to avoid discomfort and protect ourselves. But the energy generated by the experience gets trapped inside. Our bodies become a storehouse for negative imprints.

Armoring is an instinctual process that protects us against what we believe are dangerous sexual feelings. Unfortunately, this repeated tightening has the undesirable side effect of stopping the flow of signals from the nervous system, life-giving fluids, and vital energy.

When armoring persists, it deadens the constricted tissues. They become rigidly locked in place, becoming stiff instead of soft, pliant, and supple the way nature intended.

The genitals are as subject to armoring as any other part of the body — maybe even more because sexuality is subject to intense fear, guilt, and judgment from social conditioning, not to mention the devastating impact of sexual abuse. Our sexual frustrations, failures, and wounds leave their emotional and psychological energy traces in these vulnerable tissues.

THE EFFECTS OF ARMORING

How does armoring create sexual resistance? Here are the major impacts:

BLOCKED ENERGY FLOWS

As we've said, we all need the natural respiration of our energies. When tissues are armored, our channels are blocked, and life force doesn't flow.

Blockages prevent sexual messages from reaching our most powerful sex organ—the brain—which can then decrease, limit, or even stop our ability to feel pleasure. Worse, we don't have access to the energy that fuels love, creativity, inspired action, and spiritual connection.

HEALTH EFFECTS

The tension deposited deeply inside our bodies suppresses all of our physical systems. Who knows how much our health truly suffers? Permanent tension and stiffness restrict our vital feelings of desire, attraction, and arousal. Studies have indicated that armoring may affect the menstrual cycle and cause repeated vaginal irritation and urinary tract infections.

SELF-PROTECTION

Because armoring is a self-protective mechanism, it cuts us off from enjoyable experiences as well as from reliving the past traumas. It chokes off spontaneity and makes us feel threatened by what should be fun. It can make us uncomfortable talking about sex and our bodies, as well as asking for what we want in bed. It even stifles us from showing or feeling affection.

SEXUAL INHIBITIONS

When our genitals or other related parts of the body are armored, we can't totally immerse ourselves in our sensations and merge physically with our beloved. Our sexual channels can even shut down entirely. When blocked, protected, and inhibited, we need stronger and stronger stimulation to break through these shells and feel satisfied. As much as we favor any practice that brings pleasure, we believe it's entrenched armoring that causes some people to crave violence, painful intercourse, sadomasochism, and other kinky practices.

PERFORMANCE PRESSURE AND ANXIETY

When we're armored against pain, we may generate expectations that create performance pressure. Awakening sexual energy can stir up self-doubts and fears carried since childhood. We can experience internal tensions like worrying if we'll be any good at lovemaking. Will he or she like what we do? Will we be able to do it right, maintain an erection, or have an orgasm? Instead of enjoying the pleasure of the moment, our anxieties shift our attention to the future, putting unnecessary pressure on the vagina and penis.

BODY JUDGMENT

When our tissues hold onto old negative energy, our natural tendency is to disapprove of what appears to be the source of our pain—the body. Instead of appreciating the body, we judge our appearance, weight, and shape according to unrealistic social standards. Instead of loving and accepting the vehicle that allows us to live and enjoy pleasure, we condemn it. As a result, our sexual body often is subjected to the most vehement negativity. We repress our instinctive forces of nature to feel, enjoy, and procreate, generating increasingly resistant energy that feeds our armoring.

EMOTIONAL INSTABILITY

Old energy stored in the tissues is life force that lives on regardless of how hard we try to suppress it. It's like a deeply buried battery which can produce a shock but perpetually keeps recharging. These discharges can take the form of emotional outbursts or deeply ingrained negative attitudes that make little rational sense. Conventional hot frenzied sex can re-stimulate old wounds and cause volatile fights or an explosive catharsis seemingly without provocation. The pent-up pressure can trigger fantasies, past images, and repressed memories. When your lover is armored, even good-natured sexual play can evoke any number of emotions to the surface without explanation, such as anger, jealousy, rage, fear, sadness, withdrawal, pain, hurt, or depression.

Armored sex is like making love with the ghost of Christmas past. It's a form of powerful resistance expressed physically. When stored negative imprints are triggered, you may not enjoy your present. Because of dormant and stagnant energy, your zest for life can be diminished.

The more you resist, the stronger your armoring—and the more you resist. You then live in a perpetual self-reinforcing cycle of inhibition—a downward spiral that takes you further and further away from your innate blissful nature.

♣ What sexual resistances are you aware of?

♣ Is there anything about your body that might lead you to think there is some physical armoring? This might manifest as tightness of muscles and joints or as pain or skin eruptions.

♣ Is there any childhood or adult trauma from which your body might be trying to protect you?

HEALING

THERAPEUTIC MASSAGE

Unfortunately, our genital areas rarely experience the kind of healing that can melt armoring, such as sensitive massage or loving without a sexual goal.

Even the minority of the population that get enough lovemaking don't receive adequate nurturing touch. During sex, our genitals are more likely to be subjected to the heated demands of pent-up sexual desire.

You know already that we advocate passionate sex, but we also advocate healing touch for the genitals. In the coming pages, you'll learn this kind of massage for yourself and with your partner.

G-SPOT HEALING MASSAGE

This chapter culminates in one vital practice designed to be repeated as often as needed to melt all the resistance stored in a woman's vagina. This healing method uses vaginal and G-spot massage to contact and quickly move through old issues that prevent the exuberant enjoyment of sex and life.

Our cultural conditioning urges us to live in our heads, repress our feelings, and play down pleasure. This healing method urges you to get into your body and feel as much as you can in order to expand your capacity for pleasure. Instead of playing it safe to protect yourself, it guides you to take some risks and enjoy yourself as you do.

By using the healing methods that follow, you can experience:

♣ The free flow of orgasmic energy that lies dormant.

♣ Less pain, numb, or sore spots in the genital tissues.

- ♣ Greater sensitivity and aliveness in the vagina.
- ♣ Decreased vulnerability and intensity of old emotions.
- ♣ Increased sense of trust and stronger feelings of love.
- ♣ More open energy channels, allowing freer sexual expression.
- ♣ Orgasmic energy streaming through the body.
- ♣ Full-body multiple and extended orgasms, as well as the goal of this book — female ejaculation.

THE DRAWBACK OF FIGHT OR FLIGHT

Instead of focusing on problems, you can heal through the committed pursuit of pleasure. As you learn to open your energy channels, it's natural to bump into and work through any resistance that gets in the way.

When you have a problem, psychologists say you have two basic alternatives: flight or fight. If you deny the problem, try to run away, or put your head in the sand, nothing changes until it bites you. Avoiding old memories that continue to torment you adds strength to your resistance by letting the negative energy fester. If you choose to do battle with your demons, at least you're actively aware of the issues.

The shortcoming of this two-sided view is that regardless of your choice, you're being controlled by the problem. Running toward or away from a problem causes your mind to focus on it. This, of course, gives the problem more strength.

LAW OF ATTRACTION

If you keep pushing yourself to experience pleasure, the healing properties of your life force energy flow will dissolve your blocks, discomforts, and resistances. Whatever helps to make your orgasmic energy flow is the very thing that will burn away the impeding blockages and allow you to experience new heights of pleasure and ecstasy.

In other words, make love, and heal thyself. Wouldn't you rather heal through pleasure than regurgitating old hurts?

LIGHTEN UP AND HEAL

You move through your resistances by removing negative imprints and replacing them with pleasurable ones. By pursuing pleasure and opening to receive it, you clear emotional blocks and release stored energy.

It's as if the weight of resistance is lifted from your pleasure balloon, allowing it to expand more easily. Once cleared, your sensuality reawakens, and you feel a powerful resurgence of aliveness, vibrancy, desire, spontaneity, playfulness, creativity, and joy. You'll regain the potential for quick and easy orgasm or, when you choose, for continued building of passion to reach for ejaculation.

YOU CAN LEARN TO HEAL EACH OTHER

Pursuing pleasure in a healthy loving relationship is a healing path open to us all. Sometimes, when you're making love with yourself or another, old emotions and images surface. Pleasure can trigger stored pain and anger that is years or decades old. Releasing tension is a good thing, though it may be awkward, uncomfortable, or even painful at the time. If this happens to you, we recommend that you continue lovemaking with as much awareness and communication as you can muster. Then, recognize you need to schedule some dedicated healing sessions as soon as possible.

By carefully studying the instructions in the practices that follow, you can help each other release body armoring and sexual resistance.

Some might say only trained professionals should attempt this kind of G-spot healing massage. We believe that through love and awareness, whatever you do will help. You may release some energy that makes you uncomfortable for a short time, but our philosophy is that it's better to trigger this energy sooner rather than later.

SOMETIMES THERAPY IS NEEDED TO BREAKTHROUGH

When old negative energies are released through sexual healing, the pursuit of pleasure rapidly accelerates. But sometimes, resistance is so strongly embedded that beginning is impossible or traumatic.

If either the giver or receiver is unwilling to enter into vagina healing, or you find the process hopelessly stuck, professional therapy may be helpful. This is especially true for those with traumatic histories.

With graduate degrees and years of private practice in psychology and personal growth, we'd be the first to admit that in some cases, do-it-yourself healing doesn't work. Sometimes, the scars of sexual wounding, trauma, and abuse run so deep that eroding them gradually isn't practical or enjoyable. So, if you feel that help is needed, be gentle with yourself, and seek out a professional.

- Do you feel open to pursuing pleasure as a source of personal and sexual healing?

- If you don't feel open, what is getting in the way? Beliefs? Doubts?

- Do you have concerns or questions about the process of healing?

VAGINAL HEALING GUIDELINES

"Sexual healing ... can happen through pleasure and delight much more easily than they can through 'working' on a problem."

— MARGOT ANAND, *THE ART OF SEXUAL ECSTASY*

PARTNERS ARE ESSENTIAL DURING HEALING

Sexual healing through vaginal massage may need to be repeated a number of times to remove the layers of distress. The faster you go, the more painful it may be. So, there's no rush. Cleanse the vagina a little at a time, and soon, you'll arrive where you've always wanted to be.

G-spot healing requires a dedicated team effort between giver and receiver functioning as equals. You both have a vital role in the process.

You are likely to run into problems or conflict if one of you takes full control while the other remains passive. The woman in the receiving role must take responsibility for guiding the giver for optimum progress. The giver needs to respond to the woman's guidance. You need to work together proactively to create a circle of energy that's stronger than either one of you could produce alone.

To ensure that you're acting as partners pulling together, we recommend that you only conduct the practice described below as an intentional healing session, not as a knee jerk reaction to resistance or purely for pleasure.

Communication between giver and receiver is essential. If something is troubling either of you, bring it up. If either of you gets an idea or becomes concerned about anything, mention it immediately. Remember that you're both doing the best you can at each moment. Operate from a place of love, respect, and appreciation for yourself and each other. Sexual healing comes through surrender more than anything else. It takes courage, trust, and mutual support.

GUIDELINES FOR BOTH GIVER AND RECEIVER

- ♣ Stay as present as you can, tune into each other, and connect your energies. This is more important than technique.

- ♣ Always stay relaxed. If you become anxious, simply breathe until you calm down.

- ♣ You can't get it wrong. Whatever you do from a place of love will move things forward.

- ♣ Don't try to be perfect. Approach this practice as playful children exploring a new game.

- ♣ Focus more on the process than any immediate outcome. Release expectations that create performance pressure.

- ♣ Remember that the way out is the way through. The process that turned on discomfort, emotion, or pain from old memories is what will turn it off.

- ♣ You don't have to do everything at once. Start slowly, and learn as you go.

- ♣ If you need to do so, come back to the process again and again. Discharge as much old energy as the receiver can stand each time.

- ♣ If the receiver feels as if she can't go any further at any point, don't push her. Let her choose to move forward or take a break.

- ♣ Agree on a signal word or motion that will cause you both to immediately terminate whatever you're doing. Perhaps the word "stop!" or palms facing the giver will work.

- ♣ Let go of your goals for immediate breakthrough. Surrender to whatever happens each time, and be open to multiple sessions.

Healing takes as long as it takes. It may take several contacts to awaken and release old energy that's been hidden for years.

GUIDELINES FOR THE GIVER

Giver, here is your job description. We don't refer to this role as "healer" because the receiver actually heals herself. But you do have a vital function to perform that can assist her in letting go of resistance.

If you choose to help your beloved heal sexual resistance, be sure you decide to accept the role of giver freely, willingly, and for sincere reasons. Don't expect anything in return right away, or ever for that matter.

Offer your heart in total service to her. This is a privilege that you're entrusted with, and it's the height of intimacy. Accept this role from a purely loving space because you want to give, not because you need to gratify your ego or satisfy yourself sexually.

Here are some guidelines specifically for givers:

- ♣ Let go of your own needs. Follow the receiver's energy, not your own urges. Let her indications of readiness be your guide to begin, continue, and shift.

- ♣ Be fully present, hold the space, and share this rare transformation with your beloved. Remember that your selfless loving presence is your most precious contribution.

- ♣ Do everything possible to create a safe environment. The receiver must feel in control at all times.

- ♣ Be gentle, and always use tender loving care.

- ♣ Approach the vagina with reverence, respect, and a sense of awe. Remember that you're being given a sacred trust.

- ♣ Keep the process going, and support the receiver as long as she's willing and able.

- ♣ Facilitate the healing process by doing whatever you can to make her clearing work as easy and painless as possible.

- ♣ Act as a neutral sounding board for whatever the receiver needs to say. Acknowledge her feelings, and express understanding and empathy.

- ♣ If strong emotional reactions surface, realize you're not the real target. Just breathe, relax, and let them pass.

- ♣ Remember that you don't have to fix the receiver. Her consciousness does that, so just remain present through her process.

- ♣ Don't feel guilty for producing discomfort through vaginal massage. Stored negative energy is what creates that.

- Don't be scared. Giving isn't hard to do if you simply have the desire to help and follow the directions below. If you can't get over the initial natural nervousness, we urge you to see a therapist for assistance before proceeding.

- Be as selflessly present as you can in each moment. Maintain eye contact, listen attentively, and be supportive.

- Do whatever you can to make the receiver feel secure, which includes maintaining strict confidentiality about what happens.

- Make a strong emotional connection with your partner without penis involvement. The penis can act as a powerful re-stimulator of old resistance forcing the process to accelerate more quickly than the receiver can comfortably handle.

- Get permission before making any major changes. Don't penetrate the vagina or move dramatically without alerting her and receiving her okay.

- Be supportive, encouraging, and show her how much you care. Reassure her with statements like "You're doing great," "I'm right here for you," or "Take as long as you need."

- Healing is not deliberately designed to sexually arouse the receiver, but it sometimes happens. If so, gently steer the process back to healing without changing your focus to lovemaking.

- Continually check in with yes/no questions to stay in close communication with the receiver.

- Make sure *you* are always as comfortable as possible by alerting the receiver and shifting your position if needed. If you become tired or tense, it may distract your partner.

- If the going gets tough, don't run away. Honor your receiver's stated boundaries, and respect any spontaneous limitations that crop up.

- Before you begin, bathe, clean your hands, and cut your nails. If you have sores or rough spots, wear latex gloves.

- Resolve outside pressures, and empty your bladder before you begin in order to be fully present.

QTIP (QUIT TAKING IT PERSONALLY)

Resistance may take the form of strong emotions directed at the giver. It's possible the receiver may direct frustration, criticism, blame, or anger at you and what you're doing.

If it happens, resist the urge to defend yourself. Recognize that the receiver's mind is somewhere else. It isn't your current beloved who's attacking you, but someone else from long ago. She's acting out of powerful forces buried deep inside as a result of traumatic incidents. Energy imprints can actually control behavior when they resurface.

To the best of your ability, follow the QTIP guideline: Quit Taking It Personally.

Giver, here are a few suggestions that can help you stay present and not get triggered yourself into negativity:

- Excuse the receiver if she temporarily forgets to lovingly ask for what she wants or forgets to appreciate what you're offering her.

- Just accept whatever the receiver says without taking it inside and judging her or you.

- Release your partner's energy using the four cornerstones of supreme bliss, and visualize the energy streaming through your body into the ground.

- If you can't maintain your composure, gently ask for a break. If you have to interrupt the process, she probably hasn't released all of the old energy. You'll need more patience, and she'll need more healing in the future. But it's better to try again later than it is to create a rift between you now.

In the long run, as long as the two of you recover your balance, no harm is done. It just means there is more healing work ahead. If it becomes an issue between you that prevents future sessions, you might want to find a therapist to help you through the rough spots.

EXERCISE: DISCUSSION QUESTIONS ABOUT THE GIVER'S ROLE

- Do you, the giver, have any concerns about your ability to follow the guidelines?

- Do you have anything you want to discuss with the receiver about what you have just read?

- Do you, the receiver, have anything you want to discuss or add about the descriptions you have just read?

GUIDELINES FOR THE RECEIVER

Whatever resistance, pain, or wounding you carry with you, underneath it, there's nothing wrong with you. Accept yourself, love yourself, and forgive yourself. Decide to move on with your life, heal yourself with your beloved's assistance, and create as much sacred pleasure as you can.

Your job as receiver is to let go of the past by focusing on your body now. If strong emotional reactions occur, let them be. Don't suppress the feelings or memories. Confront what comes up now, or it will continue to make unwelcome visits and inhibit your ability to experience pleasure.

By allowing deep love to enter your G-spot, you can let go of old buried memories and emotions and expand your potential for ecstasy. For some women, it's the only way they can open to experience female ejaculation. Here's how you can encourage this to happen:

- ♣ Choose to receive healing freely, willingly, and for sincere reasons, not because of outside pressure.

- ♣ Be sure you feel comfortable receiving from the giver you choose. Don't let just anyone act as your giver.

- ♣ Ask for whatever you need to relax, trust, and feel safe.

- ♣ Let feelings of love enter your body, mind, and spirit through your vagina.

- ♣ Just feel. You don't have to do anything. Focus on your feelings and body sensations in order to increase your capacity to feel even more.

- ♣ Allow whatever you experience to happen — tears, words, and screams are all okay. You may also use the four cornerstones of supreme bliss to ground yourself if you discover you are numbing out from the experience.

- ♣ Don't insist on understanding what you experience if it's confusing. Simply feel whatever energy you can now without analysis or explanation. You don't have to understand in order to heal.

- ♣ Don't actively seek to escape, tune out, go numb, or distract yourself. If you have any of these impulses, let your giver know immediately.

- ♣ If you're willing, share and fully express any old memories that come up regardless of how embarrassing, anxiety-producing, or vulnerable they make you feel. Of course, if it's too difficult for you, don't share them.

♣ As much as you're able, be kind to your giver. Offer gratitude, accept his or her boundaries, and forgive any limitations.

HOW TO START RECEIVING

When you're ready to begin the process, here are some additional guidelines:

♣ Prepare by bathing, beautifying, and dressing sensuously.

♣ Make your general intentions clear without specifying any specific goals for each session.

♣ Look inside, and voice any boundaries you feel without hesitation or guilt. This might include body parts or actions that you want to be off-limits.

♣ Only give permission for your giver to enter or start when you're ready.

♣ Move and dance on your giver's fingers to aid the healing process.

♣ Stay as present as you can by clearing your mind, relaxing, and remembering to breathe.

♣ Make requests of the giver using the Feedback Cycle: 1) acknowledge something that's working, 2) ask for something different, and 3) appreciate the change.

♣ Be as responsive as you can, giving verbal and non-verbal clues about what you're experiencing in each moment.

♣ Massage your clitoris yourself any time you want to add energy and pleasure to what you're feeling inside your vagina.

♣ Use the four cornerstones of supreme bliss, including PC pumps, pelvic rocking, visualization, and sounds to move the energy you encounter.

♣ Talk about any emotions, memories, or images that come up.

♣ Afterwards, relax and let the changes integrate within you instead of rushing off to work or some other stimulating activity.

YOU DON'T HAVE TO DO IT ALL AT ONCE

Don't expect to blow through all of your resistance in one fell swoop, but you can get a long way in one session. It takes lots of powerful energy to block the free flow of intrinsic life forces like sexuality and self-love. That's why this work is often draining and energizing at the same time. You may not be up to confronting everything at once, no matter how hard you try.

Healing is often like peeling an onion. Take off the skin with too many layers at once and you won't be able to hold back the tears. Instead, plan on peeling one layer at a time.

Sexual healing, or even lovemaking, can trigger unexplained images, repressed memories, wild fantasies, and even birth traumas. When old energy first gets contacted, a torrent of confusion may tumble out, as if you suddenly released a plug on a backed-up drain. This is why we have advised you to accept whatever surfaces without having to understand, analyze, or solve it. Just let it be, and move on with the process.

EXERCISE: DISCUSSION QUESTIONS ABOUT THE RECEIVER'S ROLE

- ♠ Do you have any doubts or concerns about the guidelines, or is there anything you want to add to them?

- ♠ Has anything gotten in your way in the past that prevented you from releasing old wounds and staying present during sexual experiences?

- ♠ Giver, do you have any questions about the receiver's role that you want to discuss?

CATHARSIS TRIGGERED

Though it's unlikely, touching on severe wounding may trigger an emotional catharsis. This could take the form of long bouts of intense crying, irrational and overwhelming emotional outbursts, or even hyperventilation that causes numbness and tingling in the receiver's hands.

We firmly believe that however difficult, strong, and explosive the immediate reaction may be, it's better that the block has been contacted and the energy has begun to flow.

Remember, the tried and true therapy maxims:

The way out is the way through, and

What turns it on turns it off.

Many of our personal and professional experiences have confirmed the truth of these statements. If you can stay cool and keep the process going, whatever triggered the reaction will also discharge the energy.

Nevertheless, these upheavals can have an enormous impact on you. So, we want to offer you a pressure relief valve to bail out if you feel you need it.

SAFETY VALVES OR GROUNDING TECHNIQUES

If catharsis continues for more than ten minutes, consider using this safety valve process. When the giver judges that the receiver has processed as much pain as she can handle in one session, follow these steps:

1 Say "As soon as you're ready, take a deep breath, and hold it." This may take awhile and require multiple requests.

2 When she takes her breath, say "As soon as you're ready, exhale, and take another deep breath in your belly." Repeat if necessary.

3 When she begins to calm down, suggest gently but repeatedly that she relax and continue to breathe slowly.

4 Suggest that she let the energy drain out of her body and visualize it going into the earth.

5 Suggest she imagine that her spinal cord is energetically extending down into the earth and wrapping around a huge boulder. This visualization often creates a feeling of calm.

As giver, it's important that you maintain intense presence and eye contact while you witness your beloved's dramatic experience. Don't push her to resume the healing right away but know that you'll undoubtedly have to reconnect with the intense memory in another healing session. Most importantly, be certain that she will be okay. And giver, don't forget to breathe slowly and deeply to stay grounded yourself. It can be emotional for you to watch someone you love experience such intense emotions.

EXERCISE: CATHARSIS DISCUSSION QUESTIONS

⚓ Receiver, do you have any concerns about the possibility of having a powerful emotional reaction?

⚓ Are there any issues of trust (of self or other) that need to be verbalized?

⚓ Giver, what do you understand is your response if your lover has a cathartic (emotional) reaction? If you have any doubt, review the sections above.

THE VAGINAL HEALING PRACTICE

DYNAMICS OF VAGINAL HEALING

The vaginal healing process itself is a simple touching practice that allows full consciousness to return to all parts of the vagina, especially the G-spot. The giver slowly and gently massages around and inside the vagina to reopen communication channels within the receiver.

The tissue of a healthy vagina should be soft, supple, and vibrantly alive with sensation. A healthy G-spot can produce amazing amounts of pleasure. When armored, however, the tissue hardens and loses its ability to flow sexual energy.

This vaginal healing massage returns that life simply by touching softly and pressing gently where armoring needs to be released, and this is often most intense around the G-spot. The real work is done by the receiver as she focuses her awareness wherever she's touched.

The giver touches everywhere around and within the vagina, gradually approaching the G-spot and letting the receiver feel the life flowing to and from healthy tissues. Sometimes, the giver will contact a "hot spot" when the receiver reports some discomfort.

HOT SPOTS

A hot spot is an armored place that stores old energy, revealed by negative sensations when touched. Hot spots can be tense, sore, hard, tender, painful, numb, or — as the name implies — they may burn. Sometimes, the energy is so compacted that it feels like a hard nodule under the skin.

When a hot spot is found, the giver simply holds while the receiver breathes into the area until the negative energy dissipates.

Though this experience may be unpleasant, hot spots are a blessing. They provide an exact window into what needs to be healed to open the receiver's channels to the unrestricted flow of sexual pleasure. After the stored energy is released, pleasure, orgasm, ecstatic states, and ejaculation are much more easily accessed.

Areas of discomfort shift from session to session and from time to time within each session. It's as if blockages are fluid enough to hide from the light of touch and resurface elsewhere. So, approach each healing time as a unique moment without expectation or plan. Just accept what's there, and deal with it as it arises.

Though it might happen of its own accord, vaginal healing isn't about getting excited or having an orgasm. It's about rediscovering and awakening a woman's capacity for G-spot pleasure and ejaculation.

Below is the full instruction for the vagina healing practice.

PRACTICE: VAGINAL HEALING

1. PREPARE WITH THE FIVE S'S

Supplies, Showering, Setting, Stretching, and Settling.

Discuss Partnering Questions — desires, concerns, boundaries — in the moment. Agree on any signals or alert words.

2. HEALING MASSAGE

Giver, direct heart energy to your hands. Give your beloved a soft, slow, sensuous massage to bring her more into her body, relax her, and open her sensual energy channels. Tenderly attend to her whole body. Encourage her to give suggestions about what feels best. You can use oil for anything external if she would like.

Before moving on, be sure to work the tissues surrounding the vagina. Massage as deeply as the receiver is willing to experience, loosen the muscles and tendons around her genitals, working her PC wherever you contact it, including her butt, thighs, and pelvis.

3. IS THE VAGINA READY?

Pay attention to your beloved's breathing, sounds, hip movements, and vaginal lubrication to determine when the vagina is ready to be approached. You may also ask her directly.

This is the best time to check your preparations. Do you have all of your props handy? Do either of you need to empty your bladder or bowels again? Are you in the best position for G-spot massage? (See the G-spot massage chapter if you've forgotten.) Do you have enough towels underneath her in case she ejaculates?

4. APPROACH THE VAGINA

Ask something like "May I touch your vagina?" When she answers "yes," begin by placing one hand over her vagina, the other hand on her heart, and looking deeply into her eyes. This is a wonderful time for verbally admiring her beauty, including her vagina, and professing your love.

Approach her vagina with love and respect, gently stroking the vulva. When she's ready, stroke her clitoris as well. Soft and slow is your aim, especially at first. If she wants, let the receiver take your hand and demonstrate how she likes her mound, lips, and clitoris stimulated.

Hopefully, this vulva massage will be pleasurable and awaken her sexual juices, but your aim is not to continue until orgasm.

5. ENTRY

Giver, ask if she's ready for you to enter her vagina by asking her directly. Assure her that you're there for her at all times by maintaining frequent eye contact without looking away.

When you have permission, wipe any oil off the hand you plan to use inside. Put on a latex glove now, if needed. Liberally douse your fingers with lots of water-based lubricant. Starting with the third finger is a non-threatening beginning.

Place your fingertip inside the vagina's inner lips without penetrating. Just hold at first. Then, say "Let's try up and down," and slowly and gently stroke the vagina's lips. Next, say "Let's try circles," and move your fingertip around the inner lips without any sudden, jarring or jabbing motions. There's no hurry!

6. PROBING

Now, warn your beloved that you're going deeper, and gently insert your finger inside the vagina's mouth halfway to the first finger joint. Just rest a moment. Then, press upward gently into the tissues and ask, "Do you feel my finger?" Increase the pressure gradually until she does, and then ask, "How does it feel there?" Remember, you're probing, not arousing.

As long as there's no discomfort from your finger, continue exploring the vagina's tissues in the same way, stopping at the hour positions of the clock. (12:00 means up toward her belly, 6:00 means down toward her butt.) Step-by-step, rotate one way as far as you can and then the other. You may need to move your body or even smoothly switch fingers to reach each of the 12 positions. Don't forget to alert her before you make any major movements.

7. HEALING

The core of vaginal healing is to discover any "hot spots," tissues inside the vagina that need healing. You'll recognize them when the receiver reports tension, numbness, tenderness, soreness, pain, burning, or a bruised feeling. The giver may feel throbbing, heat, or a hard nodule.

Giver, when you contact a hot spot, stop probing and hold with a steady pressure. Go just deep enough for your partner to feel the soreness or numbness. Don't try to force old energy out of the tissue by pressing or squeezing as hard as you can.

Ask the receiver, "Describe the sensation. Breathe into it. Is any image, memory, or emotion coming up?"

Receiver, focus on the sensations in your vagina, and imagine your breath flooding them. Do your best to stay with your feelings while reporting to your giver as they change.

Giver, encourage the receiver to continue by saying things like, "Good job; continue" and "You're doing great."

Remember to be patient. Do your best to avoid distractions and interruptions to the clearing process. Just allow the energy to discharge.

She may need to yell, scream, or make other loud sounds to encourage the energy to move. As it dissipates, the vagina's tissue may feel hot, even burning. While this continues, which may be two to five minutes until a full release takes place, continue holding and breathing. You can tell when the hot spot is discharged because the sensations will subside, and the area will feel lighter. Usually, the receiver will feel great afterward.

Giver, you may want to explore the vicinity of the initial hot spot to clear out related sensitive areas.

When a hot spot is cleared and the sensations are gone, continue probing the other clock positions. Spend some time enjoying the pleasurable places that you contacted. Remember to focus on the ultimate goal of the whole experience — pleasure.

8. DEEPER

Once you've probed the 12 hours of the clock just inside the vagina's mouth, it's time to go deeper, warning her each step of the way.

Giver, insert your finger all the way to its first joint. Probe the clock positions as you did before, stopping and healing any hot spots you contact.

Then, go deeper into the vagina, half a finger joint at a time. If you both like, test a straight versus a crooked finger, different fingers, or more than one finger at a time, as well as other strokes from the G-spot massage chapter.

The G-spot often holds the most intense resistance. As you go deeper, be especially alert for hot spots between 11:00 and 1:00 o'clock, where you feel the urethral sponge swell and roughen. If the receiver feels the urge to empty her bladder, stop, and breathe together until the sensation subsides.

As you reach deeply enough to feel bones from the inside, press against her tailbone, sacrum, and pubic bone while testing for hot spots. Don't forget to probe behind the pubic bone and on all sides of the cervix. If your fingers aren't long enough, you may need to use a sex toy to reach everywhere inside the vagina.

If you discover hot spots holding a great amount of pain, don't try to release them all in one session. Continue only as long as the receiver remains comfortable. Then, come back for more healing later.

9. PLEASURE DOWN

When you agree that you've done enough clearing for one session, consider ending on a high note. Since pleasure is your ultimate aim, it's wonderful to fill the energy vacuum that hot spots can leave behind with good feelings.

Giver, ask your beloved, "Would you like to shift our attention to pleasure in preparation for ending?" If she answers "yes," begin focusing on the most pleasurable areas of the vagina. Use G-spot massage strokes, and include clitoris stroking if she desires.

Encourage the four cornerstones of supreme bliss to cleanse her energy channels and spread the ecstasy throughout her body. Orgasm is a sweet way to seal the entire vaginal healing experience, but it isn't necessary or essential, especially if she isn't in the mood after an intense healing experience.

Giver, when you sense your beloved has had enough, warn her with "If it's okay with you, I'm going to withdraw my hand from your vagina." Then, do so slowly. Don't break the connection suddenly.

Smoothly cover the vulva with your hand right after exiting. Maintaining eye contact, place your other hand on your beloved's heart, and breathe together. Giver, cover your partner with a blanket. If she wants, lie in each other's arms, spoon, hug, comfort, or cradle her body. Lie together in silence, or sweetly share the experience while holding each other.

10. CLOSING

When you're ready to end the practice, close your sacred space. You can discuss what happened if the two of you prefer, or you can wait until later after things have settled.

You can also bathe together, but be sure to drink lots of water. We encourage the receiver not to run off and do something right away. Relax, and allow the process to unfold of its own accord.

AFTERTHOUGHTS

It's possible that the first healing session may reveal little. Maybe during the second or later session, the receiver will be relaxed enough to allow her hidden traumas to be experienced through vaginal healing massage. This is an intuitive call. If she believes additional sessions may be useful, go with it, but never try to talk her into it or out of it. If you run into reluctant hot spots, the following practice provides a powerful method for addressing them.

PRACTICE: HEALING HOT SPOTS

This practice can be added into a vagina healing session if you find a hot spot that doesn't seem to release or remain cleared. If you set up a separate session to focus on specific hot spots, don't simply dive into the vagina until the receiver is relaxed, settles into body sensations, and opens her energy channels.

The more skilled the receiver is at using the four cornerstones of breath, sound, movement, and presence, the more powerful the cleansing will be, and the deeper the breaths, the more she'll be able to release. This is why a vital part of vaginal healing is for the receiver to breathe into numb, sore, or burning spots, especially in the face of strong emotions, to encourage energy release.

To speed up the healing process, use the four cornerstones in the face of any strong emotions or cathartic reactions. Recognize that venting, screaming, thrashing, sobbing, or anger are prompted by earlier traumas that have been awakened. Work together to clear the energy, and the force of the imprint will cease to have any affect on the receiver.

The stronger the emotional reaction of the receiver, the more vital that the receiver breathe and that the giver remain present with eye contact.

1. PREPARE WITH THE FIVE S'S

Supplies, Showering, Setting, Stretching, and Settling.

Discuss Partnering Questions — desires, concerns, boundaries — in the moment. Agree on any signals or alert words.

2. STIMULATING

Caress your partner's whole body, long and sensuously, with oil if she wants. Begin without focusing on the most erogenous zones. As she heats up, concentrate more on her breasts and other powerful external trigger spots. Don't forget to ask permission before touching the vagina and clitoris. Be sure to use your communication skills to stay in touch and flow together. Continue stimulation until the receiver is highly aroused and wet.

3. PROBING THE VAGINA

Giver, with permission, approach and enter the vagina as described in the previous vagina healing practice steps 3 through 6.

Use slow penetration, rotating through the clock positions as you did before. You can't assume that the landscape of hot spots inside the vagina will be the same as the last time, but if you return to work some affected areas that weren't completely cleared, you may want to move toward them more quickly than before. For example, you could enter one finger joint at a time instead of one-half and stop at only 6 positions around the clock instead of 12.

4. BREATHING INTO HOT SPOTS

Giver, when you contact a hot spot, guide your beloved to use the four cornerstones by saying, "Breathe into my finger. Move your pelvis around as you want. Make sounds that express what you're feeling. I'm here to support you."

5. FLOW ENERGY

Receiver, make sounds that seem to describe what you're feeling — loud, guttural, animal. These will encourage the energy flow. Visualize the painful energy flowing out along with your exhalation. You can even use PC pumps to exercise the affected areas.

6. ENCOURAGE THE FLOW

Giver, you can assist the energy release by breathing and sounding along with your partner.

7. PLEASURE DOWN

When you agree that you've done enough clearing for one session, consider ending on a high note as discussed in the previous practice if the receiver desires. Focus on the most pleasurable areas of the vagina with the four cornerstones. Orgasm is a sweet way to seal the entire vagina healing experience, but it isn't necessary.

When you're finished, withdraw slowly. Then, cover the vulva with one hand and the receiver's heart with your other hand. Cover her with a blanket. If she desires, lie in each other's arms, spoon, hug, comfort, or cradle her body. Lie together in silence, or sweetly share the experience while holding each other.

8. CLOSING

When you're ready to end the practice, close your sacred space. You can discuss what happened if you prefer, or you can wait until later after things have settled. If you choose, bathe together, but be sure to drink lots of water. We encourage the receiver not to run off to do something right away. Relax, and allow the process to unfold of its own accord.

Ecstasy is your birthright. Each of us came into this world knowing how to feel ecstatic just by breathing. The practices in this chapter can help you release blocks and inhibitions by experiencing and increasing the flow of orgasmic energy. This is the best way we know to experience a full, ecstatic sexual life, including that wonderful flow of fluid we call female ejaculation.

CHAPTER 7

ECSTATIC STATES

*"The essential thing is not to chase after ecstasy.
It arises naturally if your presence in the world
remains relaxed, without goals and constraints —
free, opened, and light."*

— FROM *TANTRIC QUEST* BY DANIEL ODIER

YOU'RE HERE FOR ECSTASY

MORE OPTIONS

Besides achieving female ejaculation, the purpose of this book is to offer you more options for sensational ecstasy. Certainly, you could just try more fiddling and diddling or simple "friction sex." But more often than not, untrained male lovers push for more and stronger stimulation, only to ejaculate too soon. Their women feel that something's missing. Or worse, they feel used. Isn't there something more?

Yes, there is. This chapter is about using your G-spot to create higher levels of ecstasy.

Ecstasy is intense joy, delight, and elated bliss. An extraordinary elevation of the spirit by overwhelming emotion so intense that you're carried away beyond the reach of rational thoughts and ordinary impressions.

PUMP YOUR PLEASURE BALLOON

We're going to use sexual friction for sure, but you're going to learn to include awakening the heart, the mind, the emotions, and the spirit. You're going to learn to open your subtle energy system to these powerful physical life forces. In this way, you'll enliven your body and mind and connect more deeply with your beloved.

We're going to teach you to create increasingly more physical excitement using G-spot play while juicing up other zones, including the clitoris. To get there, we cultivate extended pleasure instead of focusing on orgasm as the climax of the performance. That doesn't mean that you won't experience intense orgasms in the process.

How does this seeming contradiction occur? You experience the highest levels of ecstasy when you're completely relaxed in a high state of arousal. Concentrating, aiming, and pushing for the Big O prevents this. So, as we've explained, if you savor every last bit of sensation, the orgasm will come to you.

You're going to be actively playing with your pleasure balloon, that imaginary energy bubble inside you that limits and controls your capacity to feel. At rest, your pleasure balloon is collapsed around your genitals. As you get excited, your balloon expands.

Instead of letting sexual arousal build quickly and explode locally, you're going to learn to pump the energy into your pleasure balloon. The more you do this, the lighter you'll feel, and the higher you'll float.

By the way, the more you practice, the bigger your bubble will stretch. The more you exercise your pleasure balloon, the more flexible it becomes, the easier it expands, and the larger it can get. This means that you feel more and get higher and higher. Literally, the sky's the limit.

UNDERSTANDING ORGASM

How do scientists define orgasm (as if you need a definition)? When you become sexually aroused, your sensitive zones swell with blood, your muscles tense, and your breathing deepens and speeds up as your heart rate increases. Orgasm occurs when that muscle tension is released at the peak of excitement accompanied by pulsations in your pelvis. Masters and Johnson found about 12 contractions within 10 seconds was the norm. Then, your metabolism slowly returns to normal.

Does that fit with your experience? We bet you could add to that clinical description very colorfully. Scientists often forget to mention that it also feels great, uplifts your emotions, stops time, alters your consciousness, and creates an intimate merging with your beloved and sometimes, the whole universe. Let's not forget that it makes you healthier, too.

If we're not going to push for orgasms, why should you care about understanding them in greater depth?

To most people, successful sex means having one or more great orgasms. Sadly, many women struggle with climaxing, especially during intercourse. Having spent years trying to help women come during intercourse, Somraj can attest to that. As we noted before, many men have their climax too soon for their partners to be satisfied.

PLAYING WITH ORGASMIC ENERGY

Because most lovers don't understand how to cultivate, circulate, and conserve the energy of orgasm, this chapter was born. When you learn how to play with orgasmic energy, you can make it last, feel it all over your body, and let it take you higher and higher. Then you'll feel as if you're having full-body climaxes over and over continuously. We often call this the O-Zone.

When we first started to work with orgasmic energy during the mid-90s, neither of us were multi-orgasmic. Like many other women, Jeffre's orgasms required effort. It took too much work to go for more than one. She was never aware of ejaculating. Like most men, Somraj couldn't separate orgasm from ejaculation, so he usually came rather quickly.

Realizing how much we were missing gave us strong motivation to learn about pleasure, ecstasy, and orgasm. Dancing in this powerful sexual life force is an art form. It's the highest form of intimacy, personal creativity, and self-love.

NORMAL SEX

With "normal" sex, we usually go for maximum turn-on until we quickly explode in a blaze of glory. Then, relaxation returns for awhile until the biological forces build up again. Men take awhile to recover. The average is 19 minutes in young men, and it gets progressively longer as they age. Some women also need to recover after an explosive clitoral orgasm.

Although the explosion feels good, hasty men often roll over immediately after sex and leave their partners wanting more. The promise of orgasmic energy is that you can both reach ecstatic states that feel sensationally better and last and last. The average "normal" lover doesn't have any idea what they're missing.

Don't push for the release of energy, but savor every drop. Conserve and cherish it, spreading it around your body just the way you would roll a sip of expensive aged wine around your mouth. That's where the ecstasy lies, beyond the G-spot, and what this chapter will teach you.

EXERCISE: ORGASM DISCUSSION QUESTIONS

- ♣ How would you describe your orgasms? How do they feel?

- ♣ How do you typically orgasm?

- ♣ How satisfying are your orgasms and peaks of ecstasy?

THE SCIENTIFIC HISTORY OF ORGASM

ORGASMIC HISTORY STARTING WITH FREUD

First, let's review the modern history of orgasm. Whether you know it or not, you've undoubtedly been conditioned by some of these myths and you're certainly affected by these physiological facts.

We bet you know lots about Sigmund Freud who developed psychoanalysis in Vienna before World War II. Freud believed that all of our neuroses stem from sex. Whether you agree or not, at least he brought to the public's attention that the mind is the most powerful sex organ. When it blocks pleasure, sex isn't anywhere near as good as the original designer intended.

Freud believed that women could experience orgasm from clitoral or vaginal stimulation. Unfortunately, he had to go further and say that vaginal orgasms were better, in that they represented the orgasm of the emotionally mature woman. Therefore, he believed that clitoral orgasms were immature and somehow lesser.

Do you feel less mature when you experience great pleasure from stimulation of your clitoris? We hope not.

Many studies we've seen substantiate that 75% of women don't experience vaginal orgasm. Was Freud telling the vast majority of women that they should feel less worthy because their clitoris pleasure is second class?

Of course, we believe all pleasure is a divine gift. Our personal and professional opinion is that clitoris and internal G-spot orgasms are simply different, not better or less evolved.

It doesn't take a rocket scientist or member of the upper class to create and receive any kind of pleasure. Whatever feels good is good in your mind.

THE GOOD AND BAD NEWS ABOUT THE WONDERFUL MR. KINSEY

Freud's orgasm theory wasn't officially challenged until the pioneering behavioral work by Alfred Kinsey in the 1950s. His team interviewed thousands and thousands of people to uncover the realities of modern sexual play rather than just theory.

We have Alfred to thank for the first scientific validation of a wide range of erotic activities. Though Kinsey's efforts did swing the pendulum away from the vaginal-only orgasm camp, his methods unfortunately contained a serious procedural error.

He didn't want to be accused of "fiddling" with his research subjects, so his team of gynecologists tested female erogenous zones with a device similar to a Q-tip. Aside from the fact that this doesn't sound very sexually arousing, we know something today that Alfred didn't.

Yes, the clitoris responds to soft touch and friction like his Q-tip device could easily create. But the vagina doesn't. Most of the deep recesses of the vagina only respond to pressure, something that Kinsey's little Q-tip thingie wasn't designed to produce (in contrast to men's big thingies, which are designed to produce pressure).

MASTERS AND JOHNSON BROKE REAL SEXUAL GROUND

A decade later, Masters and Johnson did a great service to our sexual lives in their groundbreaking 1960s studies of people having sex in the laboratory. They more clearly defined orgasm and gave us the well-known four-stage model for sexual play: excitement, plateau, orgasm, and resolution.

It's too bad that they based some of their research methods on Kinsey's findings. One of their primary criteria for selecting lovers for their study was that the women had to be capable of masturbating to orgasm. So, they left out women who responded differently and concluded that the clitoris alone was responsible for orgasm in women.

Undoubtedly, they studied couples untrained in the ancient arts of love. Without knowing how to manage energy buildup, circulation, and exchange, they worked exclusively with a limited view of sexuality which, in Freud's words, was immature.

All scientists are limited by their own world view. How can you ask questions about something that you know nothing about?

ENTER THE FIRST DR. G

While all of this was going on, the G-spot was mostly ignored. More than two decades earlier, Ernst Gräfenberg, the German gynecologist, wrote his famous 1950 article about the highly erogenous zone on the upper wall of the vagina. He recognized the tissue was erectile and could produce powerful orgasms—even ejaculation.

Today, we know this is true for many women. We believe that most women can learn to enjoy these sensational sexual experiences through the practices in this book. But from what we've read, Kinsey, Masters, and Johnson, along with the great majority of modern sexologists, ignored Gräfenberg's findings.

EXERCISE: TYPES OF ORGASM DISCUSSION QUESTIONS

- What were your very first experiences of orgasm like?
- What kind of orgasms do you usually have today?
- How are they different from your first experiences?

PUTTING THE G-SPOT ON THE MAP

In 1982, Alice Kahn Ladas, Beverly Whipple, and John D. Perry published *The G-Spot and Other Discoveries About Human Sexuality.* Their still best-selling book and its media acclaim firmly established this erogenous zone as a "spot."

In a recent email, John D. Perry discussed the use of the term "spot":

> *"We toyed with several alternatives, such as 'Area,' 'Zone,' etc. and decided that all of them had both advantages and disadvantages. 'Spot' was a compromise between the lesser of many poor choices. What makes it difficult is that, not only is it different in different women, but it changes over the course of time within the same person. On top of that, there is no comparable organ with which to label it. Always bear in mind that 'G Spot' is a 'sexological' term. The correct anatomical term is 'Human Female Prostate'..."*

Whatever you call the clitoris, the vagina, or the G-spot, we just hope you accept your and your lover's body like the Star Trek movie, "The Undiscovered Country." Play, explore, and titillate whatever turns you on. That's our scientific position.

OTHER ORGASM THEORIES

In the 1970s, sexologists Irving and Josephine Singer did their part to resolve (or add to) the orgasm controversy by identifying three types of female orgasm: clitoral, uterine, and blended (a blend of the other two.) They were the first to report on the deep vaginal orgasms presumably caused by the jostling of the cervix, the opening to the womb at the top of the vagina.

The Singers found that different muscles and feelings were involved. In response to this, Ladas, Whipple, and Perry developed the two-nerve theory, claiming that different nerves feeding the clitoris and the inner recesses of the vagina and the uterus account for the reports of different kinds of orgasms. We thank them all for identifying different physiological pathways and introducing the idea of blending various sources of sensation.

There are other theories of orgasm out there. The continuum proposal theorizes that there's a spectrum of climaxes triggered by the clitoris at one end and the uterus at the other. Some believe the truth is closer to a model of overlapping spheres, which counteracts the linear male-centric mindset of most sexuality research. Foremost among them are Jennifer and Laura Berman who wrote *For Women Only*.

CLASSIFYING ORGASM

We included the history of orgasm because we thought it might provoke some introspection and motivation to learn more. But, frankly, we're not very interested in the scientific categorization of what brings us pleasure. These theories are just that—ideas that can only provide a vague approximation of what's really going on inside our bodies, minds, and spirits.

The whole body and your most sensitive tissues are interconnected anyway. Different nerves feed the clitoris and the vagina, creating orgasms that sometimes feel different. Playing with different models can help you understand what's happening inside yourself when you're getting really juiced up. Then, you can take responsibility and guide your own pleasure. By knowing what the possibilities are, you can better guide your partner to reach higher realms of ecstasy.

STAIRWAYS TO HEAVEN

Margot Anand is fond of saying: "There are as many kinds of orgasms as stars in the sky."

We know there are a myriad of different orgasms. No doubt, different folks experience them in different ways. Instead of classifying them, we want to explore different physical pathways to orgasm with the clitoris, the vagina, the penis, and the G-spot. With many of these pathways, lovers can experience single, multiple, and extended orgasms and reach the continuous state of climax we call the O-Zone.

Imagine having your most powerful triggers creatively loved while you're in the throes of extended peak pleasure. The long slow buildup and the rhythms of peaking and plateauing are well worth the trip.

While we're on the subject, let's not forget that many experience the same kind of climaxes in the heart, the head, or the other subtle energy centers we call chakras. Jeffre recently had her first thumb orgasm when her hand was being sucked after a long, full-body peaking experience.

PHYSICAL PATHWAYS TO ORGASM

"Before I understood how to open with you, I tried giving you orgasms so I knew I was a good lover. But now, all I want is your surrender. I want your heart's pleasure to ripple through your open body and saturate my life with your love. Your body's openness to love's flow draws me into you, and through your heart's surrender, I am opened to the love that lives as the universe. Whether you have an orgasm or not while we make love, your body's trust and devotional openness is my secret doorway to love's deepest bliss."

— FROM *DEAR LOVER* BY DAVID DEIDA

THAT EXPLOSIVE BLAZE OF GLORY

You probably experience sex the way most people do—as tension release. The average lover builds up sexual tension in the body when they get turned on. Untrained lovers too often treat lovemaking as a way to relieve this pressure. These mini-explosions release energy quickly in a few seconds of pleasure, sometimes with a big wet spot of the male seminal variety.

There's nothing wrong with a hot quickie now and then. You know we revere pleasure in all its forms. It's just that explosive orgasm, especially for men when accompanied by ejaculation, often drains lovers of their vital energy, not to mention their interest or ability in continuing sexual play.

Of course, if you've ever had an earth-shattering mind-blowing consciousness-altering explosion, you'll surely enjoy repeating it. So, before we consider transcendent experiences, we're going to directly celebrate the pathways to explosive climax.

TREAT THE CLITORIS RIGHT — IT'S WORTH IT!

How many lovers struggle with achieving just a single orgasm? Women often struggle to have one. Many men work hard to control themselves to prevent squirting too soon, so that their partner can reach the peak at least once. We can't count the number of clients of each gender who couldn't achieve orgasm anymore after they had started to take new medications.

In this journey to higher ecstasy, you can achieve great benefits by studying your patterns, pathways, and triggers of sexual climax. Both men and women can more easily experience orgasm and ejaculation, separate the two, and choose which they want when.

Though women can experience orgasm in many ways, clitoris stimulation is typically the fast track to one or more releases. We agree with Kinsey and Masters and Johnson that this is the primary sexual arousal pathway most women receive. It has the densest nerves, responds quickly, and is easily accessible. During self-pleasuring, oral play, and even most intercourse, the clitoris plays the major part.

One drawback to clitoris play is that having the correct approach is crucial. Many a clitoris is shy, hiding under its protective hood, making it difficult to discover. Many are super-sensitive, so much so that direct contact too soon can be shocking and even painful.

THE SYMPTOMS OF EXPLOSIVE ORGASMS

Don't get us wrong. Clitoris play is wonderful and a vital part of love-play because it's been known to spark fabulous orgasms. But let's look deeper into the mechanics of a clitoris-induced explosion.

Orgasm occurs when muscle tension is released at the peak of excitement accompanied by about a dozen pulsating involuntary muscle contractions in your pelvis. Your face, arms, legs, stomach, and butt contract. Your skin suddenly gets flushed so that you're suffused with warmth all over. Suddenly, it feels as if everything stops.

As you're overwhelmed with an intense flood of sexual pleasure, you lose touch with the outside world for a moment.

SINGLE CLITORIS-GASMS

The single female clitoris-induced orgasm lasts from 4 to 19 seconds and is accompanied by rhythmic, rapid one-second clenches of the outer third of the vagina, the part nearest the opening. The PC muscles, which surround the vagina's walls an inch or two inside the opening, tighten and pulsate.

In contrast, the deep portion of the vagina tents during this kind of orgasm, enlarging its inner two-thirds and lifting up into the body along with the uterus. It feels as if a finger or penis inserted deep inside the vagina is being squeezed at the outside end, while the inside or top of the vagina noticeably loosens and widens.

Some describe clitoral orgasms as intense and others not so much. Many report orgasms can be achieved quicker with clitoris play than with intercourse. Though clitoris orgasms can be intense and spread throughout the body, women often describe them as more superficial than deeper G-spot climaxes.

After an orgasm, the clitoris may retract and once again hide under its hood. If you found the clitoris sensitive at the start of play, you'll be amazed at how much more delicate your contact has to be after orgasm. That is, if it can stand to be touched at all for a while.

PRACTICE: SOLO CLITORAL ORGASM

In earlier practices we encouraged you to simply explore and find out what feels good. There, we guided you to play with all the pleasure you could conjure. Here, we encourage you to go even further over the top.

1. PREPARE WITH THE FIVE S'S

Supplies, Showering, Setting, Stretching, and Settling.

Arrange yourself nude in a comfortable reclining position with legs spread and propped on pillows or leaning against your bed headboard. Use pads or towels in case you're worried about soaking the bed. You may want to do this practice in front of a full-length or hand mirror.

2. TOUCHING

Begin by slowly touching, caressing, and arousing yourself. Start at the perimeter and circle toward the vagina: legs, thighs, face, neck, tummy, and breasts. Take your time and enjoy. Be sure to relax, breathe deeply, and make sounds that express what you're feeling.

3. THE VULVA

Touch your vulva gently and lovingly in the manner you prefer. As your tissues begin to warm and open, add whatever lubricant you prefer.

4. THE CLITORIS

Awaken your clitoris with soft, slow circles and straight strokes on the shaft and sides. Try clockwise and counterclockwise, up strokes, and down strokes. Vary your speed. Going too fast for too long can make your clitoris numb, so experiment with different moves, fingers, and positions to discover what feels best. Some women really like to gently squeeze the clitoris between the thumb and forefinger. Try moving your thumb and forefinger in opposite directions on the sides of the clitoris with varying speeds and pressures.

5. MORE

As you get turned on, continue experimenting by modifying the speed, pressure, and directness of your strokes on the clitoris. Always go in the direction of what feels good.

6. ORGASMIC BREATHING

Use the four cornerstones of orgasmic breathing to spread sexual energy around your body and intensify the sensations of pleasure.

7. ORGASM

Get as high as you want by filling your pleasure balloon with delicious energy. When you're ready, go for a big explosion with full consciousness. Then, relax as much as you can. Watch what happens inside and out, and enjoy!

8. CLOSING

When you decide to end your session, relax gradually, and slow down your movements. We really like the energy connection of one hand on the vagina and one hand on your heart at this point. Reflect on what worked best and what you discovered about your body.

PRACTICE: PARTNER CLITORAL ORGASM

We just adjusted the instructions of the Solo Clitoral Orgasm practice so that you may guide your lover to do all the work.

1. PREPARE WITH THE FIVE S'S

Supplies, Showering, Setting, Stretching, and Settling.

Begin with the Partnering Questions:

1. What are your intentions for this practice?

2. What are your concerns or worries?

3. What are your boundaries, both physically and psychologically?

Arrange yourself nude in a warm room and in a comfortable reclining position. Prop yourself up on pillows or lean against your bed headboard. Make sure you can spread your legs to allow your partner full access to your clitoris and vagina. Use pads or towels to guarantee that you won't worry about soaking the bed.

2. TOUCHING

Ask you lover to begin by slowly touching, caressing, and arousing you. Take your time and enjoy. Be sure to relax, breathe deeply, and make sounds that express what you're feeling. A good partner will gently remind you if you forget. The most important thing is to stay focused on your pleasure.

3. THE VULVA

Ask your giver to touch your vulva gently and lovingly. As your vagina begins to warm and open, ask your lover to add the lubricant you prefer.

4. THE CLITORIS

Ask your giver to awaken your clitoris with soft, slow circles and straight strokes on the shaft and sides. Gently and lovingly, give your lover guidance and feedback to learn your preferences for clitoris stimulation. Remember to use the Feedback Sandwich (compliment, change, acknowledge.)

5. MORE

As you become turned on, guide your giver to modify the strokes to please your clitoris to the maximum. This may include increasing the strength and speed of the stroke or varying it as you wish. Play with the speed. It can make an enormous difference!

6. ORGASMIC BREATHING

Use the four cornerstones of orgasmic breathing to spread sexual energy around your body and intensify the sensations of pleasure. The more you integrate breathing, moving, and sounding in this way, the fewer words you'll need to use to communicate to your giver. Your responses will be obvious.

7. ORGASM

Use the energy you're generating to fill your pleasure balloon and take you higher and higher. When you're ready, and with your partner's cooperation, go for a big explosion. Watch if it feels any different from the solo experience.

8. CLOSING

When you decide to end your session, relax gradually, and slow down your movements. We really like the energy connection of the giver placing one hand on the receiver's vagina, and one hand on her heart at this point.

Be sure you acknowledge each other, and give feedback. This is a time for expanding your awareness and sharing it with one another. Reflect what was best and what you discovered.

MULTIPLE EXPLOSIVE ORGASM

After a single explosive orgasm, sexual excitement declines steadily to the rest state before arousal occurs again. The release of tension is relaxing. After ejaculation, men often fall asleep, and some women have a similar reduction in their energy.

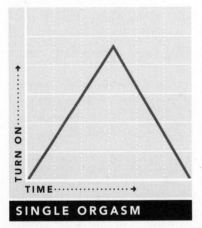

However, with the right attitude and action, there's no reason why you can't experience multiple occurrences of the single explosive orgasm. After one, your excitement will naturally dip a bit. By continuing or resuming effective stroking as soon as you're ready, you can have another climax at the same level as the previous one.

During multiple orgasm, a lover's finger or penis inside the vagina would feel about 10 seconds of contractions, then no contractions while you pause as long as you need, then another 10 seconds of contractions after more stroking, and so on. Many lovers report that this cycle can be repeated many times.

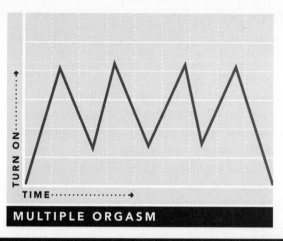

MULTIPLE ORGASM

PRACTICE: MULTIPLE CLITORAL ORGASM

You liked one. Want to go for more? Here's your chance.

1. REPEAT

Repeat steps 1 through 7 of the Solo Clitoral Orgasm Practice until you reach a big explosion.

2. CONTINUE

As soon as the receiver wants her clitoris touched again, continue stroking and massaging it. Go for another explosive experience.

3. EXPERIMENT

If multiple clitoral orgasms don't come easily for you, experiment with different uses of the four cornerstones of supreme bliss. PC pumps and energy visualizations may especially help. Test out varied strokes to see if different kinds of stimulation make multiple climaxes more possible.

4. PARTNER MULTIPLES

Teach a partner what you learned solo. Then you can lay back, relax, and enjoy a string of clitoris explosions without doing much. This is the kind of love and adoration you deserve!

5. CLOSING

Close your sacred space as appropriate. Hold each other, cuddle, spoon, etc.

VAGINAL ORGASMS

As wonderful as multiple clitoral orgasms are, climaxes induced inside the vagina have their own special qualities. The exact role that the womb and G-spot play in vaginal orgasms is still under scientific study. The Singers and others have written that pure vaginal orgasm occurs in the uterus as a result of jostling the cervix. Some believe the G-spot is the physical pathway to vaginal orgasm. Though research is still underway today, some things are clear.

G-spot orgasms are longer and deeper than those of the 10-second variety, even multiple ones. Some women report that they commonly last 45 seconds, while others say they can go on for many minutes. They involve the deep pelvic muscles including the big muscles of the uterus.

Remember that an explosive clitoral orgasm causes the deep vagina to tent, gripping near the mouth and opening up inside near the cervix.

The vagina does the opposite during G-spot orgasm. The outside third of the vagina relaxes along with the PC muscle, opening the entrance wider. The inner vaginal muscles tend to push out, closing the space. Perry and Whipple called this the "A-frame effect" in contrast to the tenting effect.

A G-spot orgasm is often accompanied by deep contractions that feel as if the uterus is pushing down toward the vagina's opening. A finger, dildo, vibrator, or penis can be forcibly ejected during this inner climax, as can the fluid that accumulates in the female prostate.

Does this help you to understand the mechanics of female ejaculation?

G-SPOT ORGASM

Here's what women say about G-spot orgasm as compared with peaks brought on through the clitoris alone.

EXTENDED

G-spot orgasms are longer with more intense contractions than clitoris climaxes. They report wave after wave of spasms that cause shaking, shuddering, and vibrating all over like nothing they've experienced otherwise.

DEEPER

G-spot orgasms are experienced far deeper. They feel as if they're pushing a woman's insides out. Some women report that it feels rooted deep within. Others describe it as whole sex erupting from heat that starts within their core and spreads throughout the whole body. One said it's like a river running loose inside.

POWERFUL

G-spot orgasms are stronger and more moving than clitoral climaxes. They're described as a complete rush, hitting the entire body like a storm or like a volcano of fireworks exploding from the vagina that makes the whole body feel like it's on fire. Some say it's like an earth-shaking tidal wave that sweeps the woman to a higher plane outside and above her body.

OVERWHELMING

Some women describe G-spot orgasm as overwhelming, causing them to lose control. They numb out, pass out, or get weak in knees. Their eyes glaze over, and they scream like never before. Some women say they lose all sense of reality, almost as if it's an out-of-body experience.

WHERE DO YOU GO AFTERWARD?

Universally, women report that the deeper orgasms resulting from vagina play are more fulfilling, as well as more emotional. That's not to say that we necessarily believe that losing touch with reality creates the best sexual experience. It's possible that these women are holding their sexual selves under tight rein. Losing their firm grip is for them a brief respite from the control they continually exert over themselves. It could also be true that the feeling of leaving the body is comforting for an instant.

We believe that it's better not to use sexual pleasure as an escape. We want you to be fully present in the experience because that's where you'll find the ecstasy.

Women report that, once they start, they don't want G-spot orgasm to stop. But when it does, they continue to feel dazed and relaxed for hours. Some report aftershocks that go on and on. Another great side benefit is that women generally want more sexual play in the immediate future.

Whatever a woman experiences, G-spot play is clearly a doorway into more powerful sensations than most women manage with external play, and certainly, playing with the clitoris doesn't eventually result in a gush of liquid. Maybe these more powerful experiences are because of the deeper pelvic nerve pathways that feed the female prostate along with the bladder, uterus, and inner PC muscle.

PRACTICE: SOLO G-SPOT ORGASM

1. PREPARE WITH THE FIVE S'S

Supplies, Showering, Setting, Stretching, and Settling.

Arrange yourself nude in a comfortable reclining position with legs spread and propped on pillows or leaning against your bed headboard. Once aroused, you'll probably have to get up on your feet or knees to reach your G-spot. Use absorbent pads or soft towels if you're worried about soaking the bed. Be sure your bladder is empty before you begin. You may want to do this practice in front of a full-length or hand mirror to watch what you're doing.

2. TOUCHING

Begin by slowly touching, caressing, and arousing yourself from the perimeter and circle toward the vagina. Caress the vulva and clitoris with your preferred lubricant. Then, lick or lubricate a finger and slowly circle around your vagina's opening, gradually going deeper inside with an in-and-out stroke. Take your time, and enjoy yourself because your G-spot may not come out to play until you're very turned on. Be sure to relax, breathe deeply, and make sounds that express what you're feeling. You might enjoy a juicy fantasy to really get your arousal going.

3. LOCATE

When you're turned on enough, you'll begin to feel places on the vagina's front wall lining become rougher and more wrinkly like corduroy. You might feel the glands harden beneath the surface somewhere between the vagina's inside end (cervix) and the urethral meatus near the vagina's mouth. With a few minutes of continued stroking, your G-spot will swell and become larger and harder, much like a clitoris or penis.

4. SQUAT

If you find you can't reach deep enough inside, or your muscles protest, continue on your knees or squat on your feet. Some experimenting may be necessary to find the most comfortable position for G-spot access. A curved dildo or vibrator can help get your G-spot aroused so that you can feel it better with your fingers.

5. PRESSURE

Gradually increase the pressure on the rough and hard spots on the vagina's front wall with in-and-out strokes about once per second. Curl your finger around the pubic bone when fully inserted, making a come-hither motion as you pull your hand out.

6. DON'T STOP

As your G-spot becomes more engorged, you may feel a sense of urgency. This is the P-Signal we talked about before—the sensation you have when you're sure you have to pee. This means you're really getting there! Remember, you just emptied your bladder. So, simply breathe and continue. The feeling will pass.

7. GO FOR IT

Use the four cornerstones of supreme bliss to intensify and spread sexual energy throughout your body. Enjoy one or more powerful G-spot orgasms. Afterward, instead of stopping abruptly, be sure to cover the vulva with your hand as you gradually cool down.

8. TOY

Whenever you decide the time is right, switch to using a vibrator or dildo for more stimulation. This is where a G-spot wand really shines, giving you leverage to apply strong pressure behind your pubic bone. Don't forget that the G-spot loves pressure!

9. CLOSING

When you decide to end your session, relax gradually, and slow down your movements. Again, we really like the energy connection of one hand on the vulva and one hand on your heart. Reflect on what you discovered and what worked best.

PRACTICE: PARTNER G-SPOT ORGASM

1. PREPARE WITH THE FIVE S'S

Supplies, Showering, Setting, Stretching, and Settling.

Begin with the Partnering Questions:

1. What are your intentions for this practice?

2. What are your concerns and worries?

3. What are your boundaries, both physically and psychologically?

Arrange yourself nude in a warm room in a comfortable reclining position and propped on pillows or leaning against your bed headboard. Make sure you can spread your legs to allow your partner full access to your clitoris and vagina. Use pads or towels to make sure you won't worry about soaking the bed.

2. TOUCHING

Ask your partner to begin by slowly touching, caressing, and arousing you from the perimeter and circling toward the vagina. Have your giver caress the vulva and clitoris with your preferred lubricant. Then, give your partner permission to insert a lubricated finger and slowly circle around the vagina's opening, gradually going deeper inside with an in-and-out stroke. Remember that you are the receiver, so you're in charge. Ask specifically for what you want, even if it differs from this description. Take your time, and enjoy yourself because your G-spot may not come out to play until you're very turned on. Be sure to relax, breathe deeply, and make sounds that express what you're feeling.

3. LOCATE

When you're aroused enough, your giver will begin to feel some places on the front wall lining of your vagina that are rougher and more wrinkly like corduroy. They might feel the glands harden beneath the surface somewhere between the vagina's inside end (cervix) and the urethral meatus near the mouth. With a few minutes of continued stroking, your G-spot will swell and become larger and harder, much like a clitoris or penis.

4. PRESSURE

Guide your partner to gently and gradually increase the pressure on the rough and hard spots on the upper wall with in-and-out strokes about once per second. Have your giver curl a finger around the pubic bone when fully inserted, making a come-hither motion as the hand is pulled out.

5. DON'T STOP

If you feel that sense of urgency, like you need to pee, remember that this is a good sign. You already emptied your bladder, so simply breathe and continue. The feeling with pass quickly.

6. GO FOR IT

Use the four cornerstones of supreme bliss to intensify and spread sexual energy throughout your body. Enjoy one or more powerful G-spot orgasms.

7. TOY

If you want, let your partner switch to using a vibrator or dildo. A specially-designed G-spot wand can really assist your lover as well, providing leverage to apply strong pressure around and behind your pubic bone. Some women like intense pressure, and it's hard for some givers to maintain that kind of pressure with fingers alone.

8. COOL DOWN

When you're ready to stop, be sure your partner knows to follow your lead so that the contact between you isn't broken abruptly. Instead, remember to have your giver cup and hold your vagina with the palm of one hand, while the other hand rests on your heart. Look into each other's eyes, and breathe together.

9. CLOSING

When you decide to end your session, relax gradually, and slow down your movements. Be sure you acknowledge each other, and give feedback. This is a time for expanding your awareness and sharing it with one another. Reflect on what you discovered and what worked best. Talk about how you both felt through the experience.

ENERGY PATHWAYS TO ORGASM

"...The solid bodies of the two lovers begin pulsating as if charged with electricity. The feeling of having solid flesh disappears. You are suddenly a pillar of vibrating energy held in exquisite balance by your lover's field of energy. This is a total orgasm of body and soul."

— FROM *TAOIST SECRETS OF LOVE* BY MANTAK CHIA

SETTING THE STAGE FOR ENERGY EXCHANGE

Not every woman opens to G-spot play quickly and easily. Early direct clitoris stimulation doesn't work for every woman either. So, blending the two can be a powerful combination. But getting there requires the consciousness of the receiver, the skill of the giver, and communication between the two.

Diving straight in to using physical techniques alone isn't the guaranteed path to sexual success. How often have you heard the complaint that men just want to pump and skip the foreplay, while women want connection, intimacy, love, or at least something more than just physical fiddling. They want sex to have meaning.

Adventuresome lovers often get hooked on stronger and stronger physical stimulation in an attempt to create more pleasure. We encourage everyone to play with all pathways that intensify sensation and orgasm. It's the addiction to stronger "external" stimulation that troubles us.

In contrast, by opening all of your senses fully, you can become more sensitive to every sensation, no matter how subtle. You can learn to immerse yourself in the most delicate whiff of pleasure, and transform it into surges of ecstasy. That's why we call S.E.X. Subtle Energy eXchange.

WHAT IS YOUR CAPACITY FOR PLEASURE?

Most everyone has ingrained limits to how much pleasure they can experience. If your pleasure balloon is restricted to the small area of your genitals, it can fill up too rapidly and explode, creating an explosive orgasm without the possibility of extended orgasm.

Somraj has always wanted it all, and he used to think he could take as much excitement as he and his lovers could muster. It was a sobering moment when he discovered that he had limits, too. Through practice, however, he has expanded his capacity for pleasure. Where will it stop, nobody knows.

By slowly stretching your pleasure balloon, more and more energy is contained without the wonderful but brief explosion that virtually pops your bubble. Slowly expand your balloon to fill your entire body with orgasmic energy, and you will feel the powerful vibrations of orgasm continuously everywhere in your body. That's the degree of pleasure you can experience if you move past your current limits.

This kind of full-body orgasm is an energy event. Truly, nothing compares to using subtle sexual energy to reach spectacular crescendos of ecstasy.

When you can circulate orgasmic energy as sexual play stimulates your erogenous zones, you don't restrict the excitement to a small confined area. Rather, you spread the electricity. When your pleasure balloon is as big as your body or even bigger, any part of your body can become as excited as your genitals during an explosive orgasm. As the sexual forces surge throughout your body, instead of seeking explosive release, they continue to surge higher and higher.

As the orgasmic energy expands, it floods your entire body with pulsing contractions and continuous wavelike vibrations. You shake all over, engulfed in surge after surge of pure liquid fire. By conserving and channeling orgasmic energy within, orgasm becomes a sacred energy event, an intimate communion, and a bonding of life forces, separate and distinct from momentary tension release.

IMPLODE, DON'T EXPLODE

With explosive orgasm, purely and simply, you discharge like a lightning bolt and lose energy. You expend the fuel that can propel you to higher states. With implosive orgasm, you still experience heart-opening, mind-blowing peaks of pleasure. You just do it in a different way.

Often, beginners resist the whole notion of giving up explosive orgasm. We understand why. They've always equated it with the peak of sexual ecstasy. We're not trying to talk you out of the best feelings you've had thus far! Enjoy explosive orgasms whenever you want. We're simply suggesting another option for you to expand your repertoire and experience potentially greater sensations.

Somraj used to feel the same way, never wanting to miss the luscious dessert after the great meal. As he became more multiply orgasmic, he changed his mind. Now, he prefers floating at peak pleasure because it's more intense than any explosive orgasm he's ever had.

But don't give up anything. Just take your time, and shift your attention to the higher, finer frequencies that you miss when you're madly humping away.

ESO

Alan and Donna Braeur's book, *ESO: How You and Your Lover Can Give Each Other Hours of Extended Sexual Orgasm*, provided another valuable piece of the orgasmic puzzle when it was published in 1983. They identified three zones or categories of orgasm: single, multiple, and extended.

While people who experience single and multiple orgasms have wonderful explosions of equivalent intensity, extended sexual orgasm is a state of continuous ecstasy that climbs endlessly. Even back in 1983, the Braeurs knew that the G-spot provides the ultimate sexual ecstasy. Clitoris play, according to them, usually only results in single or multiple explosions at the same level of pleasure.

WHAT IS EXTENDED ORGASM?

The pleasure level of extended orgasm climbs higher and higher, becoming increasingly intense and reaching amazing states of ecstasy.

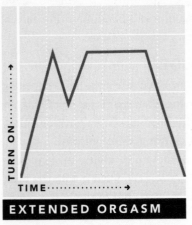

EXTENDED ORGASM

Extended orgasm usually starts with a single or multiple climax in most women and men. For men, it means an orgasm without ejaculation. Once started, lovers feel as if they're actively reaching for more and more pleasure. Later on, extended orgasm becomes self-sustaining, requiring little or no effort for the continuous slow contractions to surge for minutes or even hours.

Most women need G-spot play blended with clitoris play to enter this zone. Some sexually adept women can enter this state with clitoris or other stimulation alone or even without any sexual stimulation. But there's much more than stimulation involved, which is probably why so few women experience extended orgasm or ejaculation.

To enter this state, a woman must relax, let go, and surrender to the incredible sensations of pleasure sweeping through her. Because most women can't go from zero to 60 instantaneously, occasional leveling helps. She ramps up, absorbing pleasure that fills her balloon a little, and then floats for a moment before climbing higher with more stimulation.

Because sexual energy is conserved instead of expended, these streams of ecstasy can go on and on. It's the ultimate in recycling, the ultimate experience of prolonged peak pleasure.

THE O-ZONE

Beyond excitement, beyond single orgasm, beyond multiple climax, and even beyond extended orgasm lies the rarefied atmosphere of the O-Zone, the "Orgasm Zone."

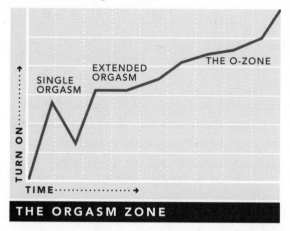

THE ORGASM ZONE

Like an Olympic gold medalist who reaches the "zone" where impossible athletic feats come effortlessly, you can reach these continuous streaming amounts of pleasure through your body. The O-Zone is a timeless place where you float without effort, and the ecstasy soars of its own accord. In this meditative, altered state of consciousness, your heart rate and blood pressure actually go down. The boundaries with your beloved disappear as you merge with the entire cosmos. Anyone who's been there will tell you that they want to stay forever, never wanting the supreme bliss to end.

A hallmark of this state is that it doesn't have to end until you choose to stop. Wonderfully, you'll stay aroused above your resting state for up to 24 hours. During this time, those delicious orgasmic contractions can easily be restarted, sometimes just by remembering them. Not only does it feel awesome, but it's good for you. You'll feel less irritable, less tense, and less stressed. You'll feel healthier, happier, more relaxed. In this rapture, it seems as if our physical limitations disappear, and we float with all boundaries dissolved.

Discuss with your partner or your journal any doubts, questions and reactions to what you've read about extended orgasm.

♠   Have you ever experienced your limit of pleasure? How did it happen?

♠   Have you ever floated in the O-Zone?

PEAKING

Let's get down to the nitty gritty of how you get to sensational ecstasy on your way to experiencing female ejaculation. The path to extended orgasm and the O-Zone doesn't focus exclusively on the best or strongest technique and how much stimulation you can create in the shortest possible time. Instead, you focus on filling your pleasure balloon.

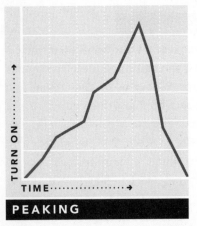

PEAKING

The first secret is peaking, which means to enjoy excitement as it rises to a high level. Then, instead of going for more and the resulting explosion, immediately change, slow down, or stop the stimulation. It's a sudden surge of turn-on that you let come back down without going over the top. Peaking just before an orgasm is, of course, great fun.

If you graph peaking, it looks like a steep ascent up a mountain followed immediately by a steep descent, which is where it got its name.

DON'T RESIST THE PEAK

Some people can't understand why you would want to back off from something that feels so good. We've answered that question extensively, haven't we? By drawing out the process, you get longer and higher pleasure. Your ultimate orgasm is more intense, often transitioning to an extended one. The more you peak, the more sexual energy you pump into your pleasure balloon.

However, so many of us try to get it over with rapidly because we're programmed with taboos, shame, and guilt about sex. Women worry that they won't have an orgasm, so they push for it at every opportunity.

If you've always pushed for as much excitement as you can muster as quickly as possible, practice peaking by yourself. Begin by ramping up and absorbing pleasure that fills your balloon a little. Then, float for a little while before climbing higher with more stimulation. This practice applies to men as well as women.

PRACTICE: SOLO PEAKING

If you have a partner, we suggest you practice Solo Peaking in front of each other. If you've never self-pleasured in front of each other, you have an exciting new experience to enjoy.

1. PREPARE WITH THE FIVE S'S

Supplies, Showering, Setting, Stretching, and Settling.

Before you begin, choose your strategy. If you aren't very skilled at peaking, we suggest you start with external stimulation on the clitoris. If you've practiced a lot, use your own judgment.

2. COMFORTABLE POSITION

Lie on your back in your most comfortable position with your knees bent and supported by a pillow, leaning against your bed headboard, or simply with your legs extended straight.

3. RELAX AND FOCUS

Begin with relaxing, conscious breathing, or full body sensual massage until you're comfortable, focused, and ready to get excited.

4. LOVEPLAY

Massage your genitals the way you enjoy it most.

5. STOPPING

As your arousal builds but before you get too close to orgasm, stop in order to back off from your first peak. When your excitement has settled down, repeat this several times.

6. SLOWING

Once you're confident about stopping, repeat the same cycle several times, but this time, simply slow down rather than stop. Change your strokes, or lighten your pressure slightly.

7. GO FOR IT

Continue as long as you want, finishing with an orgasm if you choose.

8. CLOSING

Close your sacred space, and reflect on what you discovered.

PARTNER PEAKING

Once you've enjoyed and mastered solo peaking, you'll certainly want to try it with your partner. Lovers help their partners peak by adjusting the stimulation to avoid pushing toward orgasm.

You can develop the knack to tease and tantalize long-term partners to unfathomable peaks. Practice, and improve. Don't succumb to the social conditioning that a good lover always knows exactly what to do with each new partner at each moment. That's an unrealistic expectation.

Recognize that good sex is a team game. As with the any kind of relationship intimacy, peaking works best with communication and cooperation. How do you know for sure how turned on your lover feels and what he or she wants at each moment unless you ask questions and listen?

Receivers have as much, if not more, responsibility for peaking. The receiver guides the giver with verbal feedback, by moving closer or away, getting louder or quieter, breathing deeper or shallower, or using pre-arranged cues.

PRACTICE: PARTNER PEAKING

1. PREPARE WITH THE FIVE S'S

Supplies, Showering, Setting, Stretching, and Settling.

Discuss the Partnering Questions—desires, concerns, boundaries—deciding who will receive what first. Agree on alert words or signals for slowing and stopping. If you aren't very skilled at peaking yet, we suggest you start with external stimulation on the clitoris. If you've practiced a lot, use your own judgment.

2. RELAX AND FOCUS

Begin with relaxing, conscious breathing, or full body sensual massage until the receiver is comfortable, focused, and ready to get excited.

3. LOVEPLAY

Giver, massage your partner's genitals the way she likes it. If you're unsure at any point, ask. Receivers, be supportive, positive, and helpful, and don't be shy to ask for what you want.

4. OBSERVE AND GIVE FEEDBACK

Giver, watch your partner closely for signs of rising arousal: facial expressions, swelling tissues, darkening color, changed breathing, thrusting hips, body jerks, pulsing muscles, hands pushing away, or withdrawing pelvis. At the same time, receiver, give verbal feedback about what you're feeling and about your level of arousal.

5. STOPPING

As your arousal builds but before you get too close to orgasm, give your stopping signal to back off from your first peak. Giver, immediately stop all stimulation, and resume only when asked.

6. SLOWING

After you're confident about stopping, repeat the same cycle several times, but use slowing signal this time. Giver, instead of entirely stopping, slow down, change your strokes, or lighten your pressure slightly. Closely follow what your observations, senses, and partner tell you.

7. GO FOR IT

Continue as long as you want, finishing with an orgasm if you want.

Switch roles, and repeat the practice.

Close your sacred space as appropriate, and talk about what you both discovered and felt. Finish with what feels good, perhaps hugging, holding each other, or spooning.

PLATEAUING

HOW TO PLATEAU

Once you develop the knack of peaking by slowing or stopping the external stimulation, you can move on to learning to plateau. Plateauing means:

Learning to maintain a high level of arousal without backing off.

If you picture peaking as shooting up steeply, followed by dropping down quickly, plateauing will be easy to grasp. Here, you move up to a high level of pleasure and stay there, enjoying it as long as you want.

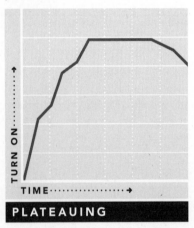

PLATEAUING

Plateauing is like mounting the steep narrow steps of a Mayan pyramid. You go slowly so that you don't slip. You stop at wider walkways, rest, and catch your breath. When you reach the top, you relax totally, float close to the sky, and simply enjoy the view.

It's possible to plateau by adjusting the outside stimulation. Try it if you haven't, and see if you like it.

We prefer and recommend learning to plateau using the four cornerstones of supreme bliss. The receiver who masters spreading orgasmic energy in this way ceases to be at the mercy of her lover. No more feelings of not being in charge of your own pleasure. When you can stream energy up and down your inner flute, you'll naturally plateau and easily transition into extended orgasm and eventually the O-Zone.

When you can circulate the energy, you can simply float on a true ecstatic high. Some call these "valley orgasms" because as their arousal curve rises higher and higher, it flattens out at steps instead of peaking up sharply.

IT'S THE RECEIVER'S JOB

As the receiver, you will manage the internal process. You're going to learn to spread even the subtlest sensations throughout your body and absorb it all in your pleasure bubble. You'll feel the slightest exciting touch on your clitoris, for example, and instead of screaming and squirming for more, you'll absorb it like a hungry pleasure sponge.

Using all four of the cornerstones are vital here—breath, sound, movement, and presence. The last is the most critical for extended orgasm. Presence is the ability to be fully in the moment, experiencing what's happening now, and letting go of any resistance that ties you to the past.

By using the four cornerstones of supreme bliss and breathing orgasmically, you'll excite all of your chakras, which store and regulate all of your energies. You will become a conduit for limitless and endless life force by breathing, moving, making sounds, and staying fully present.

RELAX

Because most lovers can't go from zero to sixty instantaneously, the receiver needs to jumpstart the meditative state by relaxing and opening fully. In short, to enter this state, the receiver must relax, let go, and surrender to the incredible sensations of pleasure sweeping through her. Easier said than done, of course.

She must focus, tune in to all sensory input, and consciously absorb sensation. Distractions can kill the mood, and the built-in resistances we all carry can easily get in the way. We're talking about negative emotions like guilt, shame, and fear that block energy, as well as thoughts and beliefs that run counter to feeling pleasure.

If a part of you hates sex because of the pain of childbirth, if intimacy conjures up the torment of failed relationships, or if you still believe that some kinds of sex are a sin, the free flow of energy will be blocked to some degree.

BREATHE YOUR WAY HIGHER

Most lovers, when very excited, pant or hold their breath. Their muscles become tense and tight. They move closer and closer to the release of explosive orgasm. The more excited they get, the more they shut off their senses and focus inward, often closing their eyes.

When this situation is coupled with the shame, guilt, and embarrassment that makes so many of us passive in bed, we end up feeling as if we don't have control over our own pleasure.

This is in stark contrast to the supreme bliss experience. You breathe slowly and deeply. You relax and undulate your body to spread the excitement. You become more and more present with your senses while fully awake, connecting with your beloved and the whole universe. You guide your experience by responding and communicating.

You rock your pelvis while you relax your other muscles, and you communicate openly while keeping all of your senses wide open. You empty the mind of extraneous distracting thoughts and visualize the energy moving within and exchanging with your partner. You use your PC muscle to pump energy up your inner flute, opening your channels to the flow of orgasmic energy.

In this manner, you bring your mind, emotions, and spirit into harmony with your body. As you can see, there's much more than stimulation involved, which is probably why so few people experience extended orgasm.

PRACTICE: SOLO PLATEAUING

You might think you've done this exercise already since it's beginning is so similar to Solo Peaking, but using the four cornerstones of supreme bliss to spread orgasmic energy while continuing to absorb pleasure is an important and vital difference. Again, even if you have a partner, we suggest you practice Solo Plateauing first.

1. PREPARE WITH THE FIVE S'S

Supplies, Showering, Setting, Stretching, and Settling.

Before you begin, choose your strategy. If you aren't very skilled at plateauing, we suggest you start with external stimulation on the clitoris. If you've practiced a lot, use your own judgment.

2. COMFORTABLE POSITION

Lie on your back in your most comfortable position with your knees bent and supported by a pillow, leaning against your bed headboard, or simply with your legs extended straight.

3. RELAX AND FOCUS

Begin with relaxing, conscious breathing, or full body sensual massage until you're comfortable, focused, and ready to get excited.

4. LOVEPLAY

Massage your genitals the way you like it best.

5. ORGASMIC BREATHING

As your arousal builds, begin breathing, moving, sounding, and moving energy using PC pumps and visualization.

6. PLATEAUING

When you feel a high level of excitement, consciously enjoy it, savor it, and relax into it. Using the components of orgasmic breathing, hold your pleasure level for a few minutes. Slow your breathing, open your eyes, move slower, moan louder, or pump your PC more to spread the energy.

7. STREAM ENERGY

Channel the energy up your inner flute, swirling it around your heart, or higher to your third eye. Can you feel the energy elsewhere in your body? Focus on it, move around it, and breathe into it to heighten the orgasmic feelings outside your genitals. If your PC muscle starts to spasm all on its own, relax and enjoy ride the wave of pleasure. You'll eventually find as you relax into a plateau, ecstatic vibrations will sweep throughout your body.

8. PEAKING

If you get too close to orgasm, feel free to stop, slow, or change what you're doing to back off from the peak. You can also open your eyes wide, relax all of your muscles, and inhale more slowly and deeply into the belly through the NOSE until your excitement drops. If your excitement keeps rising, you can also try holding your breath. Alternatively, some people report that fast panting releases energy suddenly.

9. REPEAT AND GO FOR IT

Continue as long as you want, leveling at several plateaus, and finishing with an explosive orgasm if you want.

10. CLOSING

Close your sacred space as you like, reflecting on what you discovered.

PRACTICE: PARTNER PLATEAUING

1. PREPARE WITH THE FIVE S'S

Supplies, Showering, Setting, Stretching, and Settling.

Discuss Partnering Questions — desires, concerns, boundaries — deciding who will receive what first. Agree on alert words and signals for slowing and stopping.

2. COMFORTABLE POSITION

Receiver, lie on your back in your most comfortable position: your knees bent, supported by a pillow, or with your legs simply extended straight. Giver, sit or kneel between your partner's legs or at her side. Giver comfort is as important as receiver comfort. Tension in the giver's body transmits to the receiver, so be sure to experiment until you find a position that can last awhile for both of you.

3. RELAX AND FOCUS

Begin with relaxing, conscious breathing, or full body sensual massage until the receiver is comfortable, focused, and ready to get excited.

4. LOVEPLAY

Giver, massage your partner's genitals the way she likes it best. If you're unsure at any time, ask. Carefully observe your partner for signs of rising arousal. When you see something creating great turn-on, concentrate on maintaining the same speed, pressure, and stroke without changing. Receivers, be supportive, positive, and helpful, and don't be shy to verbalize what you want.

5. ORGASMIC BREATHING

Receiver, as your arousal builds, begin breathing, moving, sounding, and moving energy using PC pumps and visualization.

6. PLATEAUING

Receiver, when you feel a high level of excitement, consciously enjoy it, savor it, and relax into it. Using the components of orgasmic breathing, hold your pleasure level for a few minutes. Slow your breathing, open your eyes, move slower, moan louder, or pump your PC more to spread the energy.

7. STREAM ENERGY

Receiver, channel the energy up your inner flute, swirling it around your heart, or higher to your third eye (the area between your brows). Can you feel the energy elsewhere in your body? Focus on it, move around it, and breathe into it to heighten the orgasmic feelings outside your genitals. If your PC muscle starts to spasm all on its own, relax, and ride the wave of pleasure. As you relax into a plateau, ecstatic vibrations will sweep throughout your body.

8. PEAKING

Receiver, if you get too close to orgasm, use slowing or stopping signals to guide the giver to back off what they're doing. You can also open your eyes wide, relax all of your muscles, and inhale more slowly and deeply into the belly through the nose until your excitement drops.

9. REPEAT AND GO FOR IT

Continue as long as you want, leveling at several plateaus, finishing with an explosive orgasm if you want. (While this book is about the steps to achieving female ejaculation, you can certainly switch roles and repeat the exercise, if you like, even if you're a heterosexual couple.)

10. CLOSING

Close your sacred space as appropriate, and discuss what you discovered. Hold each other or spoon, if you like.

BLENDED ORGASM

PLAYING IN STEREO

Short of intercourse, you've got it all now: the clitoris, G-spot, and energy to carry you to single, multiple, and extended orgasms. Play there long enough, and you'll catapult yourself into the non-stop O-Zone. We've saved the best for last: blended orgasm. This is a process of merging multiple stimulation and riding the wave. Blended orgasm originally referred to the clitoris and the vagina climaxing at the same time. We extend the term to including excitement of the lips, breasts, womb, and even the mind for that matter. Now that you've mastered supreme bliss, you can also blend energy play with any of these orgasmic triggers.

Dealing with multiple sources of pleasure is both the delight and challenge of blended orgasm. You, the receiver, will receive more sensation from more sources than you're accustomed to. Can you deal with such intense feeling? Can you handle it? Can you pump that much energy fast into your pleasure balloon? Is it flexible and expandable enough to absorb it all?

If you drop into a meditative, no-mind condition, surrender to the natural forces within your body, and let the pleasure sweep you away, you'll soar on wings of ecstasy. Delightful as it is, losing control like this can be extremely scary at first.

The giver of blended stimulation has a major challenge as well. The giver has to pay attention to two or more different actions with different responses. It's like playing two different musical instruments at the same time or like listening to two different stereo channels simultaneously.

Without confidence, experience, and total presence, a lover can't give each separate channel the attention it deserves. This is even more demanding for novice self-pleasuring when you have to both give and receive simultaneously.

BLENDING CLITORIS AND G-SPOT PLAY

Going for blended orgasm inside and outside the vagina simultaneously requires two fingers, hands, or sex toys. Inside, you can use one or more fingers on the G-spot, a dildo with or without vibration, or a G-spot wand. Outside, you have the option of using one or more fingers on the clitoris or a little vibrator.

A giver at the receiver's side with fingers inside the vagina can stimulate the clitoris with the thumb of the same hand. Skilled lovers sometimes cup the vulva and rest their palm on the clitoris or mons (the mound of the pubic bone.) This allows the other hand free to press on the receiver's pubic bone or lower abdomen covering her womb. Many women enjoy this added stimulation of the sexually responsive acupressure points on the top ridge of the pubic bone. Some report feeling delicious pressure on the G-spot from the outside. Of course, using orgasmic breathing to stream energy from the clitoris and G-spot is always available to the receiver.

PRACTICE: BLENDED FINGER PLAY

1. PREPARE WITH THE FIVE S'S

Supplies, Showering, Setting, Stretching, and Settling.

Discuss Partnering Questions—desires, concerns, and boundaries.

2. ORGASMIC BREATHING

Giver, open with a full body sensual massage. Receiver, as your arousal builds through loveplay, begin breathing, moving, sounding, and moving energy using PC pumps and visualization. Imagine that you're channeling the energy up your inner flute, swirling it around your heart, or higher to your third eye.

3. CLITORIS PLAY

Giver, massage your partner's clitoris the way she likes it best. As always, if you're not sure what she wants right now, ask. Receivers, be supportive, positive, and helpful, but don't be shy to ask for what you want. Remember the Feedback Sandwich.

4. G-SPOT PLAY

After a juicy peak or plateau, givers should switch the massage to the receiver's G-spot (with her consent, of course). Yes, we said switch! Don't do both at first. Use the strokes gradually as you learned in the G-spot massage chapter. If you're not sure what to do at any time, ask the receiver for feedback.

5. ALTERNATE

Giver, now alternate between clitoris and G-spot play, switching at natural peaks or plateaus. At each pause, encourage the receiver to relax and stream orgasmic energy throughout her body.

6. BLENDING

Giver, when the time is right, use both clitoris and G-spot massage simultaneously. Don't go to this blended massage too soon. Wait until she demands it or is responding very strongly to each single stimulation.

7. FOLLOW THE RECEIVER

Giver, follow the receiver's responses. She may guide you to help her peak, plateau, and orgasm over and over. If she chooses to continue, she may experience an extended orgasm, or she may ejaculate. Follow her lead, and stay with her.

8. SPOONING

When she chooses to wind down, maintain your attention and presence. When she's ready, connect the vulva and her heart with your hands, cuddle in a spooning position, and gently discuss what she experienced.

9. CLOSING

Close your sacred space as appropriate, acknowledging each other and your pleasure.

ORAL BLENDED PLAY

You can do the previous exercise just as well with oral stimulation of the clitoris using your mouth, lips, and tongue. Many women experience even more intense pleasure this way.

There are so many variations and options that the subject demands a book all its own. In the meantime, by using the sensitivity and skills you've developed so far, adding oral play to the clitoris should be an easy jump. Positioning the giver's body can be a challenge when combining oral and G-spot play. Experiment so that your neck doesn't stiffen up and your penetration hand doesn't cramp.

PRACTICE: BLENDED ORAL PLAY

1. PREPARE WITH THE FIVE S'S

Supplies, Showering, Setting, Stretching, and Settling.

Discuss Partnering Questions—desires, concerns, and boundaries.

2. ORGASMIC BREATHING

Giver, open with a full body sensual massage. Receiver, as your arousal builds, begin breathing, moving, sounding, and moving energy using PC pumps and visualization. Imagine channeling the energy up your inner flute, swirling it around your heart, or higher to your third eye.

3. ORAL PLAY

Giver, begin to kiss, lick, and suck your partner's clitoris and vagina the way she likes it best. If you're unsure at any time, ask. Receivers, be supportive, positive, and helpful, but don't be shy to ask for what you want. Remember to use the Feedback Sandwich.

4. G-SPOT PLAY

After a juicy peak or plateau, the giver should switch the massage to the receiver's G-spot (with her consent, of course). Use the strokes gradually as you learned in the G-spot massage chapter. If you're not sure what to do at any time, ask.

5. ALTERNATE

Giver, alternate between oral and G-spot play, switching at natural plateaus when she relaxes and streams orgasmic energy throughout her body.

6. BLENDING

Giver, when the time is right, use both oral and G-spot massage simultaneously. Don't go to this blended massage too soon. Wait until she demands it or is responding very strongly to each stimulation separately.

7. FOLLOW THE RECEIVER

Giver, follow the receiver's responses. She may guide you to help her peak, plateau, and orgasm over and over. If she chooses to continue, she may experience an extended orgasm, or she may ejaculate. Follow her lead, and stay with her.

8. SPOONING

When she chooses to wind down, maintain your attention and presence. When she's ready, connect the vulva and her heart with your hands, cuddle in a spooning position, and gently discuss what she experienced.

9. CLOSING

Close your sacred space as appropriate, acknowledging each other and your pleasure.

COMING TOGETHER?

Are things coming together for you yet? We hope so. While it may seem like a lot to do to reach your ultimate goal — female ejaculation — it's the best way we know to get there, while also discovering other intense sensations along the way.

The clitoris, the vagina, and the G-spot are all pathways to orgasm, as are other parts of your body, mind, and soul. Using orgasmic breathing can harness your sexual energy to contribute as well and can all lead you to a single climax, a series of multiple ones, an extended orgasm, and/or an ejaculation response. Blend them, and the O-Zone is just around some unexpected corners, as is that gush of liquid you're hungry for.

As the receiver, we encourage you to study your pathways to different orgasmic experiences. Discover for yourself how to fill your pleasure balloon and soar to new heights of ecstasy. How can you best use peaking and plateauing? How many and what kind of orgasms propel you into the most ecstatic of states?

If it takes you weeks, months, or even years to appreciate the ecstatic states awaiting you inside your body, that's fine. When you're ready, the next chapter expands the game to include intercourse and the prospect of sacred simultaneous orgasm. Whether you achieve ejaculation right away or not, it's certainly a fun road to travel along the way, isn't it?

CHAPTER 8

OPTIMAL POSITIONS

"Sexual behavior is to be learned with the aid of the Kama Sutra and the counsel of worthy men, experts in the art of pleasure."

— MALLINAGA VATSYAYANA, FROM *THE KAMA SUTRA*
TRANSLATED BY ALAIN DANIELOU

If you've read and played through this book chapter by chapter, you now realize that there's more to ejaculation and ecstasy than just pushing the right button. You need to prepare physically and spiritually.

The more open the receiver's energy channels, the greater the pleasure she feels, and the more likely she'll be able to ejaculate. The better the giver's partnership and more stimulating the loveplay, the more responsive her G-spot will be.

If you've experimented with the practices so far, you must realize by now that hitting your beloved's G-spot with a penis is far from automatic. As you learned with finger massage, there's an art and science to locating, engorging, and pleasuring the G-spot.

In this chapter, you'll learn how to stimulate the G-spot through intercourse. Every penis and vagina is different. Based on how his and hers interact, we'll explain how some fit better than others and what to do about the discrepancies.

Varying your sexual position is one primary method to best match the penis and the vagina to produce maximum G-spot excitement. The *Kama Sutra* is probably the best known manual that addresses this.

IF YOU'VE SKIPPED RIGHT TO THIS CHAPTER

If you've come right to this chapter, you're probably interested in making your sexual union more exciting. Great!

The bad news is that you missed how to locate and stimulate the G-spot, not to mention awakening the subtle energies laying dormant inside that can really supercharge your sexual play and lead to female ejaculation.

If you want, carry on trying out the *Kama Sutra* sex positions in this chapter. Just realize that applying the practices of the previous chapters will boost your chances of mutual pleasure enormously.

THE FAMOUS HINDU LOVE MANUAL

The *Kama Sutra* is a Hindu love manual that's nearly 2000 years old. It was translated into English by Sir Richard Burton during the 19th century. He was a much earlier nobleman with the same name as the well-known modern English actor. The *Kama Sutra* is actually just a depiction of sexual customs in India during the early centuries of the common era, but it still has much to offer us.

For example, the author, Mallinaga Vatsyayana, was very forthright about things we're too ashamed or embarrassed to talk about today—things like lovemaking positions. Though we don't know much about him, we do know that he was a sage and religious scholar who lived in Pataliputra, India between Benares and Calcutta sometime between 200 and 500 AD.

He didn't pull any punches. The *Kama Sutra* was meticulous and graphic about seduction, foreplay, sex, and love relationships, and this made it the definitive guide to sexual etiquette of the times.

PLEASURE RULES

What was the purpose of this treasured window into the past? You might have read that *Kama Sutra* means "love songs." This sounds wonderful but isn't particularly accurate.

Kama is often defined as love, a rather broad term that means various things to different people at different times. More exactly, this "kama" is about desire and pleasure derived from the senses. Kama is the enjoyment you glean from hearing, feeling, seeing, tasting, and smelling.

A simple definition of *sutra* is "rule," which would make the meaning of the title, "Rules Of Pleasure." Actually, a sutra was an aphorism, the briefest possible statement of a principle. Back then, few people could read or write. The common practice was to condense knowledge into sutras that could be easily memorized. In B.C. times, education was done mostly through oral tradition.

Vatsyayana compiled the customs of his era into these short pithy sayings. Unless you understand the history and depth behind the sutras, it's easy to misunderstand or miss his points completely.

SEX POSITIVE

Maybe our curiosity about this old book of sayings stems from living in a sex negative society, one that doesn't accept, value, or embrace erotic play as an essential part of life. To truly benefit from studying the *Kama Sutra*, you have to recognize that it was all about another time and place. Ancient India was a highly sex positive culture very foreign to ours today.

The *Kama Sutra* documented the erotic lifestyle of the most privileged upper class. Many of these people were obsessed with sex and seduction. Premarital and extramarital sex were common and accepted, as long as one followed politically correct guidelines, of course. Vatsyayana was sort of the sexual Emily Post of his time.

The good news is that Vatsyayana carefully documented the amorous practices and sexual techniques of his day. Though he did contribute his views, Vatsyayana served primarily as an editor to collect and compile the vast storehouse of Hindu erotology written by others during the previous several centuries.

WHERE DID YOU GET YOUR SEX TRAINING?

Rites of passage at the time of puberty aren't common today as they were in many ancient indigenous cultures. As part of their education, young people of Vatsyayana's time were educated in sexuality, loveplay, and the 64 arts:

> *"The preliminaries to sexual intercourse … the body of erotic treatises … considered as forming part of the practice of love."*

We expect that much of the great appeal of the *Kama Sutra* today is its down-to-earth advice about foreplay, extending the sex act, and giving maximum pleasure. Shocking, even by today's standards, the *Kama Sutra* classifies lovers according to several characteristics, including differences in sexual anatomy. Much of its advice about lovemaking revolves around sexual positions for the union of equal and unequal sized genitals.

Since it was a compendium of the customs of the times, the *Kama Sutra* also went into great detail about how to acquire a wife, how to behave once married, how to seduce other men's wives, and how to treat courtesans.

DOES SIZE COUNT?

MALE INSECURITY

It doesn't take much exposure to spam or adult websites to recognize how many modern lovers believe that size matters, especially when it comes to male sex organ.

But does it really?

A Taoist text from China declares the following about penis size:

> *"The shape and hardness with which Nature has endowed a man are only external signs. What appears internally is the skill with which he ensures that a woman derives enjoyment from his lovemaking. If a woman really cares for a man as he cares for her, then it is totally irrelevant whether his organ is long or short, thin or thick … A long, thick organ is often worse for a woman than a short thin one that is firm and hard. And a firm, hard organ that is pushed and pulled out in a crude manner is worse than a soft one that is moved about delicately and with tenderness."*

We can't begin to tell you how many women have vehemently echoed similar sentiments.

DOUBLE STANDARD

If penis size is such a subject of jokes, why don't we judge women on the size of their vaginas? The average erect penis is around 6 inches (15 centimeters). The average unexcited vagina is 4 inches deep (10 centimeters), which means that the average penis is ample enough.

How large is the opening of the average vagina? Zero. Yes, at rest, the vagina's walls press against each other. So just about any penis can make adequate contact with enough of the vagina to create the seeds of great pleasure, provided both parties know how to make the most of it.

The strength of a woman's vaginal muscles count much more than the size of her vagina. In Asia and elsewhere, skilled female lovers developed their PC muscles to the point where they could grip, milk, and make any man's penis orgasm without any other movement.

The Tamils of Southern India called this skill of vagina muscle control *pompoir*. In the Arabic world, a woman who had mastered the use of her PC muscles during sex was the "*kabbazah*" or "holder." In these places and elsewhere, female love skills were honored, respected, and revered.

If you haven't started your daily regimen of PC practices, this is a good reason to finally get going!

WHAT DOES COUNT

To be fair about the double standard, the western world does judge women on size, as the booming business in breast implants confirms. But breast size, or the size of any sexual organ, has little to do with sensitivity. So, size is rarely the determining factor in how much pleasure you receive, and size also has little to do with how much pleasure you can give.

This whole discussion demonstrates that men who think size is important often don't have a clue what counts in the sack to the average woman. We're convinced that a big part of the *Kama Sutra*'s appeal has to do with how it deals with the realities of sexual anatomy. The size and shape of the penis and vagina makes a difference in how lovemaking works between couples. If you act on the pragmatic guidelines of the *Kama Sutra*, you'll learn how to use your assets more skillfully by preparing, practicing, and compensating.

GENITAL SIZES

In India during the sixteenth century, Kalyana Malla wrote the pleasure rules documented by the *Kama Sutra* more than a thousand years earlier. It was called the *Ananga-Ranga*, or *The Stage of Love*. Both volumes define three distinct types of sex organs:

The penis is classified based on length when fully erect:

HARE Does not exceed 6 fingers long (about 5 inches)

BULL Does not exceed 9 fingers long (about 7 inches)

HORSE About 12 fingers long (about 10 inches)

The vagina is classified based on depth:

DEER 6 fingers deep (about 5 inches)

MARE 9 fingers deep (about 7 inches)

ELEPHANT 12 fingers deep (about 10 inches)

They all can work well if the owner knows how to use them to maximum advantage. Despite rumors to the contrary, no one has ever proven any correlation between genital size and physical makeup, height, strength, or race. In other words, don't expect to predict a man's penis size by the size of his feet!

MATCH GAME

Besides genital dimensions, the *Kama Sutra* classifies lovers as small, middling, or intense based on their "force of passion or carnal desire." Sex partners are also rated as rapid (short-timed), average (moderate-timed), and slow (long-timed) to come to orgasm.

The manual explained that the best match was between lovers of similar size, drive, and timing. Unfortunately, it didn't explain how would-be lovers of the time were supposed to discover these qualities for the perfect match. Do you think "test driving" was accepted in ancient India?

Since a perfect match of size, drive, and speed occurs less often than a discrepancy occurs, the *Kama Sutra*'s greatest offering is its advice about compensating for differences. It teaches how to awaken the slow and disinterested, how to lengthen loveplay for the too-quick man, and how to rekindle the fire when lost.

This Hindu love guide is probably best known for its detailed listing of sexual positions and how they can be used to adjust for genitals that don't fit perfectly.

EXERCISE: GENITAL SIZE DISCUSSION QUESTIONS

♣ My penis/vagina's size is…

♣ I would rate my level of passion as…

♣ My normal time to come to orgasm is…

WHY WE LIKE THE ULTIMATE GENITAL UNION

What we find so special about intercourse is the unifying of two energies into one. When we both have open channels that shoot orgasmic energy throughout our entire bodies with the slightest stimulation, we can connect, exchange, and reinforce each other's sensations. Through this resonance, we each magnify the force of the other's pleasure. The feedback cycle becomes a self-reinforcing loop.

Of course, the version we're all accustomed to is simply that what feels good to one feels good to the other. When he speeds up and gets really turned on, she feels it and responds in kind. This turns him on even more. When she wants to slow down and feel every millimeter of his penis caressing her vagina's, oh so delicate walls, so does he.

You probably already knew all that. We just hope reading this little reminder turned you on as much as it did us writing it.

THERE'S JUST DOING IT, AND THERE'S REALLY DOING IT

Shortly, we're going to describe all manner of contortions you can get your two bodies into during penetration. We just don't want you to forget everything we've covered so far that precedes the intercourse. Make your lovemaking an intimate event, not an athletic contest. Approach it with wonder in a gentle and sweet way. Maintain eye contact. Murmur love and appreciation often. Act as conscious partners joined together in a really fun game. Don't be shy. Be open about what you want, but talk softly and freely when you do.

Be responsive, and show what you're feeling with your breath, sounds, and movements. Spread the delicious sensations you're creating together. Share them. Alternate between giving and receiving, and prove you care by not pushing for orgasm. Instead, glide into pleasure together, and play with the energy. Enjoy your peaks of pleasure by relaxing into them. It isn't a race, so don't rush. Make it last and last.

CHANGING POSITIONS IS A DANCE

There's no such thing as the perfect position. Each has its own advantages and disadvantages, benefits and risks, uses and limitations. For one thing, bodies are different. Experiment to discover what's pleasurable for the meeting of your two unique physical forms. Your size, shape, strength, flexibility, stamina, and limitations will have lots to do with determining your favorites.

As you play with positions, consider the following:

- Are you both comfortable?
- Can you easily get into the position without hurting yourself or your partner?
- Is it relaxing, or is it tiring?
- Does it allow freedom of movement for only one of you or both of you?
- Can the dominant partner support their weight without putting too much pressure on their lover?
- Is penetration at the right depth—not too deep or shallow?
- Can you see each other and your genitals?
- Does it allow for easy communication and coordination?
- Do you both feel secure in the dominant and passive role required?
- Can you reach places you want to fondle, such as the breasts, clitoris, testicles, anus, etc.?
- Most importantly, does it feel good?

SHIFTING WHETHER YOU'RE DRIVING OR RIDING

As we get more into sex positions, it's important that you get comfortable with changing postures. Here are some suggestions:

- Learn how to easily adjust by adding variations.
- In order to shift together, develop a smooth, easy way to communicate through words, movements, gestures, or other cues.

- After shifting, resume thrusting slowly at first to see how it feels. Gradually go deeper and faster until you're sure it's working.

- Be aware of what your partner is experiencing when you want to shift so that you don't get out of sync with one another.

- Alert your lover if you need a sudden shift due to an ache, cramp, or soreness.

Make changing positions a dance that not only adds interest, variety, and new sensations, but lets you rest limbs and body parts that tire. Don't continue when either of you feel tension, but shift to relieve the stress, ache, or pain as soon as possible. Don't forget to warn your beloved first, of course.

HELPING THE PENIS TO AWAKEN THE G-SPOT

If you've completed the earlier practices and are confident you can find and excite your lover's G-spot, your next assignment — guiding his penis to do the same — should come more easily. Remember, most G-spots prefer pressure over friction, but there are guidelines for both sexes that can help you "hit the spot."

FOR MEN

- Angle your penis toward the back or front of her vagina.

- Use fast, short, or hard strokes targeted at the G-spot.

- When you find a delightful spot, hold still inside with pressure. The receiver's feedback makes this much easier.

- Alternate pressure and rocking on the G-spot.

- Hold your penis in your hand and churn it around the vagina.

- Ride up higher and grind on the top of your lover's pubic bone to press the G-spot from the outside.

WOMEN

- Move into the best position to receive maximum G-spot stimulation.

- Take charge of stroking to direct thrusts to your G-spot.

- Get on top and control rhythm, depth, angle, and length of strokes.

- Motivate your partner to respond to your suggestions with kind, supportive, and complimentary words.

- Once your G-spot is engorged, ask for short thrusts with the penis' head, sometimes punctuated with short periods of holding.

EXERCISE: INTERCOURSE DISCUSSION QUESTIONS

- What I like most while the penis is inside the vagina is...

- What I like least while the penis is inside the vagina is...

- What I would like more during intercourse is...

- What I would like less during intercourse is...

- What I've found gives me maximum G-spot stimulation is...

EQUAL RELATIONS

According to the *Kama Sutra*, the best match for lovers, called *equal relations*, is with corresponding genitals: large with large, medium with medium, and small with small.

In old Indian terms, the three possibilities are:

Hare + Deer

Bull + Mare

Horse + Elephant

With equal relations, penetration is easy. The woman doesn't need to open or contract her vagina. The man need not aspire to athletic postures to compensate for different sizes.

The *Ananga-Ranga* says: "When the proportions of both lovers are alike and equal, then satisfaction is easy to achieve. The greatest happiness consists in the correspondence of dimensions."

UNEQUAL RELATIONS

Unequal relations, according to the *Kama Sutra*, are between lovers whose genitals are of different sizes. The more unequal, the more difficult it is to achieve satisfaction.

HIGH UNION	Man one size larger than the woman
HIGHEST UNION	Largest man with smallest woman
LOW UNION	Woman one size larger than the man
LOWEST UNION	Smallest man with largest woman

Of course, these labels aren't really important. We've included them so that you'll be aware of how much compensation you need.

PREPARING FOR HIGH UNIONS

A baby is much bigger than the largest penis. Vaginas were designed to expand tremendously to allow for birth, so we know the potential exists to accommodate Highest Unions with pleasure instead of pain.

With High and Highest Unions, lubrication is of the utmost importance, however. Three of your most vital guidelines are wet, Wet, WET!

If you're a Hare Woman (smallest) or Horse Man (largest), you'll likely be in this tight lovemaking situation often. If so, be sure you use lots of commercial water-based lubricants to assist.

We believe much of the difficulty with High Unions is insufficient warm-up. This is a situation in which you definitely can't rush into a quickie. You might need up to an hour or more of ample loveplay to insure that the vagina is totally hot, open, and thoroughly engorged.

POSITIONS FOR HIGH UNIONS

In High Unions, you want to choose sexual positions and postures that allow the receiver to spread her thighs to make the vagina's inside space bigger. Makes sense, doesn't it? All you need to do is to become familiar with the positions that work best in each situation. In the next section, you'll find a large variety of wide open positions and postures that create extra room for a large penis in a small vagina.

To allow High Union penetration to be as comfortable and pleasurable as possible, consider The Receiver Position (woman on top), Transverse Position (side-to-side), the Her Legs Wide Posture of the Giver Position (man on top), and the Wide Open Posture of the Kneeling Giver Position.

PREPARING FOR LOW UNIONS

Fortunately, there are also great ways that both men and women can use to compensate for Low and Lowest Unions. They all work better after both have dedicated themselves to regular PC practices. We've already mentioned pompoir, the skill of a woman with strong vagina muscles trained for gripping and milking the penis. The better the receiver can pump her PC muscle, the better for Low Unions.

As the *Kama Sutra* states about the largest vagina: "The elephant woman contracts her sex to receive a small caliber." The *Ananga-Ranga* says that the woman must "strive to close and constrict her vagina until it holds his penis as, with a finger, opening and shutting at her pleasure, and finally acting as the hand of the girl who milks the cow. This can be learned only by long practice."

Don't worry that this long practice is a burden without reward. The stronger a woman's sexual muscles, the easier her orgasms come, the more powerful they are, and the more likely she is to ejaculate ecstatically. Worth the exercise? You bet!

Women, if you're feeling singled out, don't. This isn't sexist work. Men who build strong PC muscles can develop stronger, harder erections. With enough strength, they can apply more pressure where it counts on the G-spot. If you've ever experienced pulsing finger pressure on a G-spot, imagine that being applied by an erect penis. It sure puts a delicious bounce in your step. Again, men can receive the payoff through longer stamina, stronger orgasms, and prostate health.

POSITIONS FOR LOW UNIONS

In simple terms, when a woman's vagina is larger than the penis, use positions, postures, and variations in which she tightens her thighs. For Low Unions, avoid the wide open variations that make too much space inside. The Cow Position (rear entry), The Giver Position (man on top), and Kneeling Giver Position are some that can help.

EXERCISE: POSITION DISCUSSION QUESTIONS

🪷 My favorite position is…

🪷 My least favorite position is…

🪷 A position I've always wanted to try is…

🪷 What I am doing to strengthen my PC muscles is…

KAMA SUTRA POSITIONS

HITTING THE SPOT

We'd love for this section to tell you exactly which posture you must use to best hit your beloved's G-spot. But if you've read the book up to this point, you know that we can't. In any given lovemaking session, the following factors can influence how well his penis contacts her G-spot:

- ♣ Fit based on relative penis girth and vagina width.
- ♣ Fit based on relative penis length and vagina depth.
- ♣ His and her PC strength and tone.
- ♣ G-spot type and location.
- ♣ Erection hardness, curvature, and angle relative to his body.
- ♣ The vagina's natural angle and configuration.
- ♣ G-spot sensitivity and preferred strokes.
- ♣ Pubic bone contact between him and her.
- ♣ Location and sensitivity of her urethral meatus.
- ♣ Angle of penis entry due to chosen sexual position.

As we've said so many times, degree of excitement affects G-spot pleasure, so we can't leave loveplay, especially with regard to the clitoris, out of this equation.

Just don't give up hope! The truth is out there ... or, more accurately, in there. You just have to put on your intrepid explorer hats and experiment. Make believe you're Lewis and he's Clark (or the other way around, if you prefer).

This chapter lists all of the sexual positions and practices to test which work best for you. By being aware of the above variables while you're playing and staying in close communication with one another, you'll become your own best sex coaches.

CHOOSING SEXUAL POSITIONS AND POSTURES

There are seven basic sexual *positions:*

1 **THE RECEIVER POSITION**   (woman on top)

2 **COW POSITION**   (rear entry)

3 **TRANSVERSE POSITION**   (side-to-side)

4 **THE GIVER POSITION**   (man on top)
5 **KNEELING POSITION**   (man between her legs)
6 **YAB-YUM POSITION**   (sitting)
7 **DANCING POSITION**   (standing)

You can modify each position using multiple *variations* by moving torsos, adjusting limbs, and shifting weight. To bring some order to all of the options, we've grouped the variations of each position into several categories that we call *postures*.

The listings below contain several postures for each of the seven positions, and each posture can be changed into several variations.

Many *Kama Sutra* lovemaking positions derive from Yoga stances (asanas). Over the long term, yoga practitioners develop strong and supple bodies. That's why many of these positions are too physically demanding for the average modern lover. But it doesn't matter because there are still plenty of new and exciting alternatives for everyone.

We originally included the applicable *Kama Sutra* names for postures and variations in our listing. Because the names are strange and somewhat obscure, this made our list somewhat confusing. Since your main concern is finding the best ways for the penis to hit the G-spot with your unique anatomies in mind, we figured you wouldn't mind if we simplified things by leaving out the history.

POSITION EXPERIMENTS

Below, we describe the seven major positions, each followed by a practice. These position experiments are your chance to explore all of the intercourse arrangements that work for your bodies. These lovemaking sessions are designed to help you discover which sexual postures and variations create the best G-spot pleasure in the most comfortable way based on the combination of your unique physiques.

We recommend that during each practice, you play with one or two postures at a time. Don't try to experiment with every variation for every posture during one practice session. You will decide what you like by seeing how much pleasure you can generate, not by just going through the motions.

Plan to repeat this practice with several new options each time. Even after years of intercourse, we still find new variations that we enjoy and want to explore further.

Once you've explored everything you want, you'll know what you prefer based on the desired effect at different times. For example, on different occasions, you may want to:

- ♣ Heighten your sensation
- ♣ Slow your peaking
- ♣ Increase G-spot pressure
- ♣ Deepen your intimate connection
- ♣ Push for orgasm

ORDER OF EXPERIMENTS

What's the best order for experimenting? There's no standard. Maybe you'll want to try to reach the G-spot with some familiar postures first. Then, in later sessions you can bring in more inventive and challenging variations to find out how they feel. You may be pleasantly surprised.

While practicing different variations within a posture, give some attention to your transitions:

What flows best from one to the next?

- ♣ Do you want to gradually move into another variation that only requires a slight adjustment?
- ♣ Do you want to try something radically different to change the mood?
- ♣ Do you want to simply bask longer in the pleasure created by what you're doing right now?

As before, begin each practice session by agreeing which postures and variations you want to try.

THE RECEIVER POSITION (WOMAN ON TOP, MAN ON HIS BACK)

One of the best positions for G-spot play is with the man on his back and the woman on top facing toward him. This makes it easy for her to control the depth, angle, speed, pressure, and rhythm of the thrusting.

She can move fast, slow, deep, shallow, up and down, and side to side. The woman is in charge of extending loveplay or pushing for orgasm. She can push his legs together or apart, varying the tightness of the fit of his penis. In some variations, she can lean over to kiss him, rub her clitoris on his pubic bone, or pleasure her clitoris herself.

Because the woman is in the driver's seat, we call it The Receiver Position, since the receiver has most of the power, acts as the initiator, and her energy leads.

Many of the following postures can be varied by the man extending his legs out straight, raising his knees or hips, or bending his legs with knees open.

KNEELING FORWARD POSTURE

With the woman kneeling over her lover while facing towards his head, she can sit upright, lean forward, or lean back.

SQUATTING FORWARD POSTURE

When the woman squats over her lover while facing toward his head, she can bounce up and down with her feet on the bed or on his thighs.

LAYING FORWARD POSTURE

With the woman laying forward and facing toward the man's head, she can lay flat on top of him with her legs inside or outside of his.

SITTING ON TOP POSTURE

In the variations of this posture, the woman sits on top of the man facing toward him, away from him, or sideways with her legs on top of his body.

FACING BACKWARD POSTURE

When the woman faces backward toward the man's feet, she can sit over him or kneel while leaning forward, backward, or rocking.

PRACTICE: THE RECEIVER POSITION EXPERIMENTS

1. PREPARE WITH THE FIVE S'S

Supplies, Showering, Setting, Stretching, and Settling.

Discuss the Partnering Questions. We've suggested that you discuss which postures of The Receiver Position you want to try first. Let's say you decide to explore the Kneeling Forward and Squatting Forward Postures this time.

Agree on any signals or alert words that you want to be prepared to use.

2. LOVEPLAY

Ritually undress each other, whispering endearments and compliments as you reveal each body part. Exchange whatever loveplay excites you both. Give your beloved a soft, slow sensuous massage. Play with the penis and the vagina using your hands, mouths, and tongues. Use the four cornerstones of supreme bliss to ensure that both of your inner energy channels are hot, full, and flowing.

3. INTERCOURSE

Slowly move into lovemaking, emphasizing one of the variations of the first posture you've agreed on. Experiment with different speeds, angles, pressures, and rhythms. Stay conscious of all of your sensations. Adjust within the posture variation for maximum contact with the G-spot. Pause occasionally, communicate, and enjoy, but be willing to shift when your body or partner needs a change.

4. NEXT VARIATION

When you agree that you've fully explored the first variation and thoroughly enjoyed all its pleasures, try the others you have decided upon in the same way. Without changing your primary posture, move into different variations by adjusting your leg positions and weight distribution as described above.

5. NEXT POSTURE

When you agree that you've fully explored all of the listed variations for the posture and enjoyed them to their fullest, check in to see how you're both feeling. If you're still energetic and hot to trot, try one or two more postures in the same way. Watch that you don't rush through each variation without smelling the flowers. Remember, pleasure is your goal, not completing any agenda, and that includes ejaculation.

6. ORGASM

If you've been filling your pleasure balloons and flying higher and higher by exchanging orgasmic energy, you may come to the conclusion that loveplay doesn't require explosive orgasm for a sense of completeness. But if you want to have an orgasm or ejaculate, go for it all the way and enjoy it fully!

7. CLOSING

When you're ready to wind down, maintain intimacy physically and emotionally. When the penis is removed, cover the vulva or each other's hearts with your hands to keep your sweet connection alive. Touch each other softly and gently. If you want, talk about what you experienced, what you liked and didn't like, and what you'd like to try next time. Share your appreciation for each other. Spoon, hug, kiss, and synchronize your breathing.

COW POSITION (REAR ENTRY)

For most mammals other than humans, rear entry is the only option. Rear entry affords some of the deepest reach. Because the vagina is angled up, the deeper the penis penetrates, the greater the chance of hitting deep G-spots. The higher the man rides behind his beloved, the more he can aim at a shallow G-spot.

Rear entry postures allow a man more freedom of movement than his lover. However, the receiver can swivel, sway, and raise her butt to guide the penis to her sweetest spots. By closing or spreading her legs, she can regulate the tightness of the fit. She can also easily play with her clitoris in this position. Experiment with pillows underneath the receiver to adjust the angle of the fit.

One disadvantage of the Cow Position is that communication is more difficult. You can't see each other or maintain eye contact. Since penetration that's too deep can be painful, you also need to be careful to lengthen strokes gradually and gently.

BENT OVER POSTURE

Standing, she bends over while supporting herself with her hands on the bed or floor, or she gets on her knees and supports herself with her hands, elbows, or shoulders while he stands or kneels behind her.

FACE DOWN POSTURE

The woman lies flat on her stomach or on a pillow that rests under her hips, face down on the bed. He kneels behind her or lays flat on top of her with his legs inside or outside of hers.

SIDEWAYS POSTURE

While she's on her side, he kneels behind her or lies on his side and spoons her so that they cup each other with knees bent while he's tucked against her back.

TRANSVERSE POSITION (SIDE-TO-SIDE)

The advantage of side-to-side postures is that both lovers can vary their thrusting without the effort of supporting themselves. She doesn't have to depend on him or vice versa. The receiver's hips are free enough that she can direct the angle of thrusting to address her G-spot most directly. The man can adjust his thrusting by moving one or both of his knees up toward her. Both can lie next to each other or at right angles in order to redirect the penis toward her G-spot.

WOMAN ON BACK POSTURE

The woman lies on her back with the man lying at right angles to her with his legs intertwined with hers (the popular Scissors Position), or she can put her legs over his hips or lift her knees to her chest.

WOMAN ON SIDE POSTURE

She lies on her side with legs drawn up toward her chest while the man kneels behind her.

BOTH ON SIDES POSTURE

They face each other on their sides with their legs straight or intertwined, one over the other's hips or with him between her legs.

PRACTICE: TRANSVERSE POSITION EXPERIMENTS

1. PREPARE WITH THE FIVE S'S

2. LOVEPLAY

3. INTERCOURSE

| 4. NEXT VARIATION |
| 5. NEXT POSTURE |
| 6. ORGASM |
| 7. CLOSING |

THE GIVER POSITION (MAN ON TOP)

These postures are generally called the "Missionary Position" because it was used by the Europeans who tried to convert Polynesians when they tried to bring Christianity to the Pacific. The Polynesians thought the man on top position was funny because they so much preferred squatting lovemaking postures.

Mostly, the man superior position has wide freedom of movement, and the woman below has little. Uninventive use of the missionary position often misses the receiver's G-spot due to its typical angle of penetration.

There are adjustments for The Giver Position, however, that allow for good G-spot contact. If he holds her bottom in the air and she raises her hips with pillows, it can work well. Or she adjusts the vagina's orientation with various leg adjustments. By raising her hips, she can direct the penis to the front wall of the vagina and often to the G-spot.

HER LEGS TOGETHER POSTURE

While on top of her with her legs together, he can move his legs inside, outside, or on top of hers with his weight on his hands, elbows, or knees. These variations of the classic Missionary Position with her legs together compensate for imperfect penis-vagina fit but don't allow much opportunity to guide the penis to the G-spot.

FLANQUETTE POSTURE

The French call half-facing variations of the Missionary Position the "Flanquette." This is where his body is swiveled to one side of hers. He can put one leg between hers or both to one side, while she places one leg across his thigh.

HER LEGS WIDE POSTURE

She opens her legs wide with her knees up or down or wrapped around him as he lies on top and supports himself on his hands or elbows.

HER LEGS UP POSTURE

As the receiver raises her legs more and more, she initially directs the penis deeper, then deep against the vagina's front wall, and then further and further toward the vagina's opening. She does this by bending her legs back, raising her knees, and placing them on his chest or shoulders. For many women, this is great for G-spot play.

PRACTICE: THE GIVER POSITION EXPERIMENTS
1. PREPARE WITH THE FIVE S'S
2. LOVEPLAY
3. INTERCOURSE
4. NEXT VARIATION
5. NEXT POSTURE
6. ORGASM
7. CLOSING

KNEELING GIVER POSITION (MAN BETWEEN HER LEGS)

In these postures, the man kneels, squats, or sits between the woman's legs. With these adjustments of the old Missionary Position, different angles and depths of penetration can be reached. In almost all cases, she's on her back with her legs or hips raised.

WIDE OPEN POSTURE

To compensate for a too-tight fit, she spreads her legs with her knees or bottom up while he kneels between her legs, possibly supporting her.

HOLDING POSTURE

In these wide open variations with him kneeling, her legs hold him between her thighs with her legs in the air on either side of his waist or crossed around his back.

CHEST POSTURE

She puts one or both feet or her knees on his chest to raise her hips and adjust her orientation for maximum G-spot contact, possibly crossing her feet or knees, while he kneels before her.

SHOULDERS POSTURE

To raise her hips even higher, she puts one or both legs or feet on his shoulders, alternating them, or crossing them.

HEAD POSTURE

In these more acrobatic variations, she rests one or both feet on his head or forehead for maximum elevation.

PRACTICE: KNEELING GIVER POSITION EXPERIMENTS
1. PREPARE WITH THE FIVE S'S
2. LOVEPLAY
3. INTERCOURSE
4. NEXT VARIATION
5. NEXT POSTURE
6. ORGASM
7. CLOSING

YAB-YUM POSITION (SITTING)

Yab-yum means mother-father because the Hindu creation myth portrays the woman sitting on the man's lap with the fruits of their lovemaking dripping down and creating the universe.

Sitting lovemaking postures are some of the most intimate and energetically satisfying, but they're demanding physically. The delight of yab-yum provides great motivation to go to the gym regularly or develop greater flexibility with yoga postures.

Most sitting postures don't allow much freedom of movement, so they aren't the most likely for G-spot contact. He needs a strong and lasting erection, and she needs strong PC muscles to milk a waning penis. If both lovers have flexible hips, adjusting the angle of penis entry is possible. If he has strong PC muscles, he can apply wonderful pressure to her G-spot steadily or by tapping.

YAB-YUM POSTURE

In the classic intercourse posture, he sits in lotus position with one leg crossed over the other, half-lotus with one leg underneath and the other crossed in front, or with legs straight, while she wraps her legs around his back. Yab-yum is also fun on a chair with her facing toward him or away from him.

STRADDLING POSTURE

By kneeling, squatting, or sitting, lovers can straddle each other, approximating yab-yum by wrapping one or both legs around their partner.

RAISED POSTURE

From yab-yum or straddling, the woman holds one or both legs in her hands and raises them as he supports her leg(s) in the crooks of his elbows, or she rests them on his shoulders.

LEANING POSTURE

From yab-yum, both lovers lean back, supporting themselves with pillows or their arms, with her legs on either side of his hips or on his shoulders. Alternatively, both can rest their legs on each other's shoulders.

FURTHER BACK POSTURE

From the leaning posture, both hold each other's arms, swing to and fro, or lie flat on their backs.

PRACTICE: YAB-YUM POSITION EXPERIMENTS
1. PREPARE WITH THE FIVE S'S
2. LOVEPLAY
3. INTERCOURSE
4. NEXT VARIATION
5. NEXT POSTURE
6. ORGASM
7. CLOSING

DANCING POSITION (STANDING)

Standing postures are exciting, but they require the greatest strength and agility. Knee bending is essential for thrusting, and pelvic rocking is a must for G-spot contact. We just wouldn't put this one anywhere near the top of the list for G-spot stimulation.

Lift-off requires the greatest exertion for these postures. A reasonably strong man with a lighter woman can enjoy some ecstatic minutes standing, walking, or even dancing.

BOTH STANDING POSTURE

With both standing, they face each other and support themselves against a wall while entwined. He can also hold one of her legs against his hip.

SUSPENDED POSTURE

With both standing, the woman is suspended from his body while she sits on his joined-together hands. He can also hold her up with his hands under her thighs, or he can hold her above his waist by supporting both of her widespread legs in the crooks of his elbows.

BED OR TABLE POSTURE

She sits or lies on her back on the edge of a bed or table while he stands between her legs with her legs stretched out at his sides, wrapped around him, or high in front of him.

LOVE SWING POSTURE

One way to make the standing position more comfortable is to buy a love swing. This is basically an adjustable hammock open on one end that you suspend from the ceiling or a collapsible metal frame. The woman lies fully supported on her back with her butt at the edge of the fabric. Good love swings include stirrups for her feet and a center bar that she can grab with her hands. He can move in and out or pull her to and fro onto his penis by holding the swing's sides.

PRACTICE: DANCING POSITION EXPERIMENTS
1. PREPARE WITH THE FIVE S'S
2. LOVEPLAY
3. INTERCOURSE
4. NEXT VARIATION
5. NEXT POSTURE
6. ORGASM
7. CLOSING

KEEP ON KEEPING ON

After your initial experimentation, we urge you to repeat these practices often to keep your lovemaking fresh, alive, and creative. If you approach each intercourse session with a clear mind, open heart, and childlike exuberance, you'll have lots to play with forever, and you'll discover lots about your G-spot that might even lead to ejaculation during intercourse. Wouldn't that be a thrill?

Remember, though, that the G-spot can be quite shy. It needs to be carefully and lovingly coaxed into showing itself, and this is even truer during intercourse. As we've said on many occasions, every couple is different, every fit is unique. Let's not forget to mention emotional variables, relationship issues, and comfort in communicating about sex. Everything is open to change in the moment.

Ancient Indians weren't that interested in finding the woman's G-spot and turning her into a multiply orgasmic lover. So, their descriptions don't indicate how well they'll work for you and your partner in finding her G-spot. Only practice and your attention to sensation will answer that question for you.

We've discovered that level of turn-on and engorgement has a lot to do with how well Jeffre's G-spot is stimulated during intercourse. It isn't solely about position, but that's very important, of course.

We hope you never stop experimenting with one another. Ride with it, play with it, and thoroughly enjoy it.

CHAPTER 9

ACHIEVING FEMALE EJACULATION

"I read your article about female ejaculation. I had never heard of it until I actually did it. I attribute it to the fact that I have become relaxed with my sexuality and therefore not afraid to release. I never orgasmed when I was younger. The first time was when I was 38 (I am 42 now.) I have 'shot' up to 3 feet before, but last weekend I shocked myself and my boyfriend. He was between my legs and playing with my G-spot and clit, and I shot right at him. So much came out that he was soaked from chest to lower belly. I was embarrassed at first until I saw the glint in his eyes and the smile on his face. He LOVED It. Now I am even more relaxed with who I am."

— CATHY FROM *MEDICINE HAT*, ALBERTA, CANADA

TIME TO PUT IT ALL TOGETHER

TRY IT, YOU'LL LIKE IT

Remember the punch line from the TV ad years ago: "Try it—you'll like it?" That's how we feel about female ejaculation.

Many women are natural ejaculators. Others have taught themselves to be. But it's probably more common than you think. In one of our recent on-line surveys, two-thirds of our female visitors reported that they ejaculate.

Scientists estimate that from 10% to 40% of women are conscious of ejaculating when their G-spot swells with adequate arousal and massage. This means they can tell when they emit sexual fluids distinct from vaginal lubrication. Some dribble, some gush, some downright squirt and spray. Mostly, this happens during orgasm, but some women do it at other times, too, when they're really turned on.

IT'S TRULY WONDERFUL STUFF

Believe Jeffre when she says it's not just for show. "It's a truly ecstatic experience you don't want to miss out on!" Since the payoff in sexual ecstasy is so fantastic, you definitely want to explore your Goddess-given talent to gush.

Women who understand the gift of ejaculation relish this feeling of warm release, and their lovers swoon when showered with such an intimate gift. Somraj, for one, finds supreme delight in being doused by the nectar.

Maybe you're worried that you can't achieve ejaculation, but believe us, any woman can develop the knack. Before you're done with this chapter, you'll know exactly how to go for it, and if you've worked through the practices up to this point, your body will be primed and ready for the experience. Isn't that exciting?

WHERE TO START

Since this book is about female ejaculation, you might have been tempted to skip directly to this chapter. We applaud you for going for what you want, but it's only fair to warn you that learning female ejaculation depends on the many other things contained in prior chapters. Dribbling, squirting, and gushing is a package deal, depending on much of what came before.

You need to understand female anatomy, G-spot massage, and orgasmic response. We can't promise, but knowing about these things may be essential for you personally to be able to experience ejaculation. On the other hand, a woman with a well-trained partner who already experiences mind-blowing G-spot orgasms is already very much on the verge of gushing.

Did you know that the word *orgasm* comes from the Greek, "to swell with wetness?" That means that ejaculation is every woman's birthright. But anything worth doing is worth doing with as much pleasure as possible, which is why we strongly recommend you read the previous chapters before attempting to master female ejaculation.

On the other hand, if you're committed to trying it now, go for it with our love and support. If you don't get the hang of it quickly, you can always go back to study the skills earlier in this book.

WHY EJACULATE?

If you're a woman, why would *you* want to learn to let your waters flow? If your partner is a woman, why would you want *her* to learn?

Whether you just think it's cool, you want to experience something new, or you imagine that having continuous orgasms would be ecstatic, you're on the right track. It's just another of life's intrinsic flows. If you say "Yes!" to life, you'll probably want to say "yes" to ejaculation.

Learning to let your waters flow increases your sensitivity and enhances your pleasure. When you can surrender to the full sexual power lying dormant deep within, you free untapped reservoirs of life force. It's empowering and liberating to many women to learn to "spill their seed" and be applauded for it like guys for so long. Plus, a wet orgasm is often a great orgasm. Why not strive to have bigger, better, stronger ones if you can?

Learning to ejaculate can also help you release negative emotions trapped in your tissues that create sexual blocks and inhibitions. In fact, if you've lost interest in sex, love, and intimacy with your beloved, learning to ejaculate can be a great way to recapture those feelings.

CONTROVERSIES

Despite the conclusive evidence that the G-spot and female ejaculation exist and have been documented since the Greek Golden Age, many authorities have refused to acknowledge them. If you ask your family physician or even your gynecologist about it, you may be surprised at the negative response.

Because of this ignorance, in the modern United States, many hapless women have had completely unnecessary surgery to correct urinary incontinence. Doctors call unwanted peeing *incontinence*. It makes us sick to think of the destructive and unnecessary surgeries performed when some women are simply experiencing something that's normal, healthy, and pleasurable.

Chemical analysis has proven that female ejaculate is not urine because it contains such small amounts of urine's key components. It's sweet, thin, and chemically different.

Anyone who's been with a female ejaculator knows it has little or no odor and is mostly colorless, not yellow. It's mostly clear and sometimes has a little milky portion with a watery consistency. In fact, female ejaculate more closely resembles a thinner version of male semen, but obviously without the sperm cells.

What is it, exactly? It contains a higher level of glucose than urine. Also, it includes two components of urine, urea, and creatinine, but in much smaller concentrations. Female ejaculate also contains PSA, prostate specific antigen, and the enzyme called prostatic acid phosphatase. These last two are also found in the secretions from the male prostate.

CULTURAL CONDITIONING

While we're on the subject of history, it's interesting to consider the Batoro, an indigenous tribe in Uganda, who teach their young women to ejaculate before marriage. Batoro women who can "spray the wall" are considered to be more desirable than those who can't.

Now, that's a twist in sharp contrast to the modern western world, isn't it? Imagine having your mother, aunts, and their best friends teaching you how to have G-spot orgasms and soak the bed with wetness. It's mind-blowing, right?

The Batoro elevate sexual pleasure to a respected place in society. They believe it's good, so there is no psychological conflict associated with it. We wish modern westerners could honor their sexuality so fully. Many of our social and physical problems come from sexual ignorance and wounding early in life leading to unfulfilling sex lives, not to mention unfulfilling lives in general.

We hope your own journey toward becoming a fully sexual woman or man will allow you to be open with your children. Wouldn't it be great if all parents approached sex in a way that doesn't perpetuate their own shame and doubt? Wouldn't it be wonderful if all parents supported their children's growth, confidence, and pride in their ability to be sexual?

If you're proud of your sexuality and feel no shame about it, you will find it easier to be more frank with your children than your parents were with you.

A STORY ABOUT HOW IT REALLY SHOULD BE

The man and woman checked into the motel about three in the afternoon. The room had mirrors all around, including over the bed. A large hot tub was in the corner. They plugged in the boombox and started playing their favorite lovemaking music. After decorating the room with flowers, candles, and ample towels all over the bed, they slowly undressed for each other.

"I want to pleasure you beyond your wildest dreams," he said as he looked into her eyes. She sighed deeply and began to lightly scratch his shoulder and arm. His penis began showing signs of growth. She could feel that her vulva was already swollen, but she wanted to go slowly and savor every moment.

They opened the bottle of champagne, and he filled the two glasses with bubbly. They crawled into the tub and gazed deeply at each other. "I love you with all my heart," she whispered. His mouth opened and with wonder, he said, "My God, you're so beautiful."

After lightly bathing and laughing a lot, they dried each other off and moved over to the king-sized bed. After about an hour of stroking, light massage, delicious licking, lots of moaning, and energetic orgasms, his penis was hard as a rock. Fortunately, her vagina was very swollen and juicy and ready to be penetrated.

Looking deeply into her eyes, he slowly lowered himself, and his penis began to penetrate her. He was attentive to the speed as he carefully moved in and out. His penis entered just a little more with each stroke because he knew that was exactly what turned her on the most.

The deeper he went, the louder and louder her screams became. When he was all the way inside her, she had her next orgasm. Interspersed in her peaks and climaxes was the feeling that her waters were beginning to flow.

She was slipping into the O-Zone and found that her orgasms were coming regularly. With each orgasm, she pushed out without even thinking about it. Her partner responded by making sure his penis didn't come out all the way. With his penis at the opening of her vagina, he could feel her ejaculate warm and wet against his skin. She writhed and moaned as he moved inside all the way again.

With each orgasm, her ejaculation became more voluminous. After about ten orgasms like this, he just had to look. Being turned on visually like most guys, he wanted to see the fluid pour out of her.

The next time she had an orgasm and pushed out, he withdrew his penis all the way and watched a huge amount of ejaculate gush from her vagina and spray him. They both simultaneously exclaimed "wow" and laughed. Without much delay, he put his penis back inside her and stroked some more.

When both began to tire and feel a little hungry, they decided to take a break. Before closing, they cuddled close and whispered "sweet everythings" into each other's ears. Both of them agreed it was the hottest sex they had had in a very long time, and both knew there was more to be had after dinner. (By the way, the towels covering the bed were completely soaked.)

EXERCISE: ATTITUDE DISCUSSION QUESTIONS

♣ Do you feel you've inherited any taboos about female ejaculation? If so, what are they?

♣ Do you have any concerns about ejaculating on your partner?

♣ If you could change your attitude completely, how would you like to feel about female ejaculation?

THE ANATOMY OF FEMALE EJACULATION

DIFFERENT KINDS OF WETNESS

Female ejaculate is different than the wetness that develops when a woman gets turned on. Vaginal lubrication isn't expelled from the urethra but from other glands, including the Bartholin glands on the lower wall of the vagina. As Gräfenberg pointed out in 1950, female ejaculate appears around orgasm, not at the beginning of arousal. Even if it was thick enough, that would make it of little use as a sexual lubricant.

If you ejaculate enough, you'll be able to prove this to yourself quite quickly. You may need to add more and more lubrication from the outside as the watery fluid washes away the thicker, more slippery, friction-fighting fluids.

This has happened to us all too often. Jeffre's common practice is to squirt or dribble repeatedly during our lovemaking. As a result, her thin ejaculate washes away our preferred sexual lubricant, which we use during intercourse to reduce friction and increase sensation. Reapplying the lube is just a routine part of our lovemaking as we pause at peaks and plateaus of ecstasy.

THE FLUID COMES IN DIFFERENT WAYS

As Gräfenberg pointed out, female ejaculate gushes, squirts, or dribbles at orgasm. Our experience is that it can be a trickle, a flood of two cups, or anything in between. You may have seen videos where the woman gushes a great deal. Some of you may not become big gushers like this, but you can have a fantastic time learning how to flow your waters at your own level.

The amount of ejaculate seems to vary with age, menstrual cycle, genetic factors, diet, physical apparatus, hydration, relationship comfort, and psychological barriers. We believe that many women already ejaculate but don't know it. It's highly likely that every highly aroused woman ejaculates a bit at orgasm. But not knowing about the possibility, many aren't aware of it. They may be dribbling such a small amount of fluid that they and their partners don't notice it.

YOU JUST CAN'T SCHEDULE EVERYTHING

Some women ejaculate every time they have sex, and some experience it only with certain lovers and certain types of loveplay. Some experience it rarely, while others flow only at certain times during their monthly cycle. Once you're practiced, you'll find out what kind of an ejaculator you are.

We know ejaculators who gush repeatedly and voluminously. Some self-appointed experts declare that women will ejaculate four or five times before they're spent. It's our experience that an experienced woman can regenerate quite quickly, maybe within 30 minutes, particularly when she's in the O-Zone.

The point we're making here is that women are different from each other and from time to time. Don't try to predict when and how much you're going to expel or develop strong expectations. Performance anxiety doesn't help. On the contrary, it actually impedes the flow.

FROM WHENCE DOES IT FLOW?

Exactly where does female ejaculate come from? You've read the historical accounts that it's expelled from the urethra, which is the canal that conducts urine out of the body. It's about 1 to 1-1/2 inches (2 to 3 cm) long and lies just above the vagina's upper front wall under the skin. The opening of the urethra is just inside or slightly above the vagina's mouth.

Our friend, Dr. Gary Schubach, also known as "Doctor G," proved in his doctoral research that female ejaculate is emitted from the urethra. He studied several copious ejaculators and, by completely emptying their bladders of urine first, clearly identified ejaculate issuing from the same place as urine—the urethral opening. Even though it comes from the same place, however, don't forget that ejaculate has been proven to *not* be urine.

The entire urethral canal is surrounded by a series of up to 40 spongy little glands and ducts that carry the name *paraurethral sponge*. That's because "para" means "beside, near, or alongside." It's the paraurethral glands which make the tissue sensitive, erectile, and can secrete fluid in times of high arousal. The G-spot is a part of this tissue.

THE FEMALE PROSTATE

Because ejaculate fluid is so similar in composition to male prostatic fluid (without the sperm cells), and the genetic origin of the sponge is the same as the male prostate, sexologists today call this tissue the *female prostate.*

Foremost among them are Dr. Milan Zaviacic, a medical professor at Comenius University in Bratislava, Slovakia. In 1999, he published twenty years of studies of women's prostates documenting their nature, configuration, and emissions. As a result of his and others' research, we know that the female prostate or paraurethral sponge contributes to female ejaculate because of the unique chemicals contained in the ejaculate.

Zaviacic also documented the different configurations of these glands, most near the vagina's mouth. As a result of all of these studies, there is now a consensus that female ejaculate is the secretion of both the paraurethral glands.

EXERCISE: EJACULATION DISCUSSION QUESTIONS

- How much and how often do you ejaculate?
- What part of your urethral sponge is most sensitive and erectile?

HOW TO FEMALE EJACULATE

OUR WET STORY

Jeffre has always been a highly sexual woman and powerfully orgasmic. Since she practices and exercises frequently, she's developed extremely strong sexual muscles in her pelvis. As you've heard, the strength of these PC muscles determines the strength of a woman's orgasms and her ability to ejaculate.

In the past, Jeffre always had orgasms by pulling inward with her PC muscles. It wasn't until she saw a film about female ejaculation that she realized pulling in actually retards the ejaculation response.

She and Somraj began practicing with push-outs, consciously forcing the muscles around her vagina outward. Though it did take some dedicated practice before she learned how to let it happen, it didn't take long once she discovered this information. Then, more practice was required for her to build the confidence that she could ejaculate regularly.

Practice is an important key. The more a woman practices, the more she can depend on her response and the more easily the flow of fluid begins.

WHAT TO DO AND WHEN

As we've said, for the vast majority of women, female ejaculation doesn't occur like flipping a light switch. It takes preparation, the right mood, and a high degree of arousal. Long, sensuous loveplay and filling your pleasure balloon completely are prerequisites. Pelvic armoring that hasn't been healed can block the whole process. Using the four cornerstones of supreme bliss to spread the sexual energy throughout your body helps tremendously.

When you're really turned on, your whole vagina becomes engorged with blood, but your G-spot has to be aroused enough to be filled with fluid. Here's where the G-spot massage strokes from our G-spot massage chapter really come in handy. It's essential to apply strong pressure with these strokes where the sponge is most engorged.

P-SIGNALS

How can you know when you're ready to gush? You learn to recognize "P-Signals." We use the letter "P" because feeling the urge to pee is the initial signal that the G-spot is fully aroused and swollen. But other "P's" apply, too. An engorged Paraurethral sponge/female Prostate puts the same kind of Pressure on the neck of the urethra as a full bladder.

Understanding this feeling is vital in learning to let go and ejaculate. The sensations of the P-signal typically occur at Peaks of Pleasure but feel different than what you may be accustomed to. That's because it's activated by the Pelvic nerve, not the one that serves clitoral orgasm. (How's that for a lot of P's in this process?)

We believe that female ejaculation is instinctual, buried deep within the ancient recesses of your brainstem. To ejaculate, you have to let go of control by your conscious mind and get out of your own way. When you feel the P-signal, you need to relax and let the sensation wash over you. Often, the sensations shoot down your legs.

If you're afraid of spraying yourself, your partner, or the bed with urine, you'll never let go. That's why it's essential that you empty your bladder fully beforehand or any time it feels full. And protect your sheets or other playing surface with towels or waterproof pads.

PUSH, PUSH, PUSH

That's three P's, but once you learn to shower and gush, you'll understand that the "P" in P-signal really stands for "push out." This means the same kinds of muscle contractions that you use to empty your bladder or your bowels or to give birth. Yes, that kind of pushing!

It's not uncommon that women pee or defecate during childbirth. Many women report having the most phenomenal orgasm of their life while giving birth.

To ejaculate, ensure that you're excited enough, and simply push the fluid out at a pleasure peak. This requires flexing the PC when you get the P-signal. When you're first learning, removing the finger, toy, or penis from the vagina encourages squirting.

G-spot orgasm helps many women by creating strong deep contractions, but sexually powerful women with strong PCs can squirt without climaxing.

Can you see how female ejaculation is the culmination of everything you read earlier in this book? Now, maybe our recommendation to read the earlier chapters makes even better sense.

EXERCISE: P-SIGNAL DISCUSSION QUESTIONS

♣ Have you ever felt the P-signal?

♣ What did you think it was?

♣ What did you do when you felt it?

WITH A WILL, THERE'S A WAY

The sexual anatomy of women is deliciously intertwined and integrated. For an experienced ejaculator, gushing can happen from other sources than the G-spot. You have at least two physical channels of stimulation: the G-spot and the clitoris. The fact is that the clitoris and the vagina's outsides are fed by one nerve, while the inside of the vagina where the G-spot is located is fed by another nerve. The average woman gets more outside clitoris stimulation during sexual play than inside G-spot contact.

When this second powerful inner pathway is opened up, you'll probably experience waves of pleasure much more intense than anything you've ever felt before. This often breaks through ingrained resistance, allowing the nectar to flow. When you fully open to you sexual power, you can ejaculate from either G-spot or clitoris stimulation, or from both together.

OTHER PATHWAYS TO GUSHING

If the ejaculate comes from the G-spot, how is this possible? A highly orgasmic woman can easily spread subtle sensations to other parts of her body, building engorgement wherever she chooses. So, there are other routes to female ejaculation than the most direct pathway through the G-spot.

A little known aspect of female anatomy makes this easier to understand. The clitoris isn't simply a sensitive little bud hiding under the intersection of your outer lips a couple of inches above the vagina's mouth. The clitoris also has a shaft that extends upward toward the pubic bone, and it has legs that extend back down toward the vagina's insides. In fact, different lobes of this extensive system of erectile tissue spread to all sides of the vagina, including the G-spot.

Now, it's likely that, similar to most women, you can feel different sensations localized in different parts of this extensive super-clitoris in response to different kinds of sexual play. Of course, now we know that all of these parts are interconnected, which means you have a physical channel to spread excitement from one part of your genitals to other parts.

If you're relaxed in your sexuality with open energy channels, touching the clitoris from the outside can stimulate the G-spot on the inside, and touching the G-spot from the inside can stimulate the clitoris. If you're skilled in circulating sexual energy, this can further expand engorgement from one place to another.

With enough practice, stimulating any sensitive area can stimulate all other sexually responsive areas. Touch a breast, and the clitoris swells. Nibble an earlobe, and have an orgasm. Tap the sacrum, and ejaculate. With the build-up of enough sexual energy, you can reach the O-Zone and ascend into a state of continuous ecstasy.

Once a woman is in the O-Zone, she might ejaculate when her partner kisses her, brushes her neck, looks lovingly at her, or just whispers endearments. Wow!

POTENTIAL CHALLENGES AND HOW TO OVERCOME THEM

We've already discussed the emotional issues that can get in the way of pleasure, but physical conditions can get in the way of learning to ejaculate, too.

FEMALE DISORDERS

Female disorders that irritate or inflame your reproductive system can impede your sexual pleasure. This may include pain or discomfort due to a physical condition, such as a vaginal or urinary infection. Inflammation of the paraurethral glands is analogous to male prostatitis and may be caused by an infection. Not only is this painful, but it can get worse if not treated right away. If you're healthy, you shouldn't experience pain during G-spot massage or any attempt to ejaculate. If you do, see your gynecologist.

MEDICAL CONDITIONS

Medical conditions in other parts of your body can impede your ability to relax and enjoy sexual pleasure. This includes illnesses that sap your energy, such as the flu, or problems that cause back or hip pain. Anything that affects your nervous system's response to sexual stimulation can get in the way of pleasure, orgasm, and ejaculation.

MEDICATIONS

Medications and certain herbs that affect blood flow to your genitals or retard the nervous system can decrease your responsiveness to sex. Anti-depressants, especially, can inhibit sex drive in many people. Check with your physician if you have questions regarding the potential side effects of your particular medication.

DISEASE

As far as we know, there haven't been any studies to date linking STD (sexually transmitted disease) transmission to female ejaculation. Our greatest concern is spreading the life-threatening HIV and Hepatitis C viruses. We do know that these and other STDs are passed from one lover to another by introducing fluids into the bloodstream. It's logical to assume that there's a risk of ejaculate fluid carrying infectious organisms. We urge you to openly discuss your sex history and exchange recent STD test results with new partners. If you become aware that your partner has an infectious condition, it's best to avoid play that results in squirting. Unless you address your fears, concern about disease is a common cause of the psychological resistance that prevents people from letting go sexually.

EMOTIONAL ISSUES

While we've already outlined the emotional issues that get in the way of pleasure, let's talk about how these issues specifically relate to female ejaculation.

LETTING GO

Fear of letting go is the biggest barrier to learning to ejaculate. You have to learn to surrender in order to have that kind of gushing orgasm. If you feel that fully giving in to your sexuality is dangerous, you'll be driven to maintain tight control. You'll do much better the more you like sex and the more you like a variety of sex. Remember that there's no right or wrong, good or bad. Your body is your temple — your gift from the gods. Enjoy and experience all that you are, and don't be afraid of getting messy.

TRYING TOO HARD

"What will my lover think of me if I can't?" Trying too hard can be its own problem. When you're learning to ejaculate, there's a temptation to push out before you're aroused enough. You can end up putting too much pressure on yourself and creating performance anxiety. Let whatever happens unfold in its own time, and enjoy the ride. Maybe you won't get it the first time or even the second or third time. So what?

You can still have a great time. Once you figure it out, you have it for life, so cut yourself some slack.

PARTNER PRESSURE

"Come on, baby, spray me NOW!" Real or imagined pressure from your partner can create the kind of tension that impedes the learning process. Learning to squirt requires releasing mental stress and surrendering to orgasmic energy. Without surrendering, you'll limit your ecstasy, wet or dry. So, just let go of any kind of pressure and enjoy yourself.

RELATIONSHIP ISSUES

When you push the envelope and try something new, relationship issues often rear their ugly head, particularly when it has to do with sex. You might run into your partner's lack of patience or ability to empathize. You might also discover that you have fears that your partner will judge you sexually. It's a good idea to talk about any fears of judgment or feelings about bodily fluids and excretions. Without addressing these issues, you may find yourself unable to relax and get turned on enough to ejaculate.

Do your best to begin the process with an open, accepting, and optimistic approach. If you find that you have difficulty learning to ejaculate after half a dozen sessions, take the time to review the challenges above, as well as the chapter about healing. Most likely, the issue is psychological, but if you work with a therapist, you can probably resolve it and still enjoy the ejaculation experience.

EXERCISE: CHALLENGES DISCUSSION QUESTIONS

- ♣ If you've experienced any of these challenges in the past, how did you deal with them?

- ♣ Do you feel that any of these challenges are in your way now?

- ♣ What do you propose to do about these obstacles?

PRACTICING FEMALE EJACULATION

NECESSARY CONDITIONS FOR FEMALE EJACULATION

Have you accepted the fact that, with the right information and training, you can learn to let your feminine waters flow? We suspect if you're able to let yourself go and experience peak pleasure, you've already done it at least a little bit.

Some women get very turned on and have multiple orgasms during sexual play, yet they're not aware of ejaculating. If your sexual muscles aren't strong enough to expel ejaculate with force, it's quite possible that you're dribbling without noticing it.

Ejaculating is mechanically quite simple as long as you're ready emotionally and physically, such as getting your PC muscles in shape. It's the preparations that can sometimes be a bit demanding. And, of course, you need to be hydrated. Don't forget to drink lots of water before, during, and after.

If you are pre-orgasmic, meaning you have trouble climaxing, it's essential that you learn to have orgasms before trying ejaculation. Otherwise, you may hopelessly frustrate yourself. There's nothing wrong with you; you just haven't had the information, the space, and the safety necessary to realize your orgasmic potential. There are many great books and videos out there to assist you. We highly recommend Lonnie Barbach's *For Yourself* and videos by Betty Dodson.

Physically, you must be aroused enough that your G-spot swells with fluid. We think that explains why many women haven't found their G-spots and ejaculated fully. How turned on is enough? If your G-spot is engorged enough to be palpable, which means that you can feel it under the vagina's front wall, you're getting there. This takes time for most women. For the average woman, we're talking about a minimum of 30 minutes of loveplay, including words, kissing, stroking, oral sex, and finger stimulation of the clitoris and vagina.

You also need intense stimulation of the G-spot in order to expel fluid. As you learned in prior chapters, the G-spot responds more to firm pressure than friction. To squirt, you'll probably need to gradually work up to hard and fast stroking. Even women who commonly have G-spot orgasms with intercourse may find it difficult to ejaculate with penis penetration at first. For most women, fingers work best, particularly in the beginning. Fingers are more reliable because they can move faster, vary the firmness, and change angles more easily. Of course, each woman is different. So, expect a learning curve that involves a lot of fun experimentation! Just never forget to enjoy the journey.

Another thing to remember is that what works for you at one time may not do the trick the next time. This is why communication between partners is essential. Learning to gush is not a time for mind reading or making assumptions. Women need to learn what to do to make it happen and share that quickly with their partners, and their partners need to be willing to ask questions. In essence, female ejaculation is a team effort.

EXERCISE: EJACULATION READINESS CHECKLIST

Did you take the short quiz in the Introduction Chapter to find out how ready you are to let your feminine waters flow? How ready were you then?

For women, ejaculation is the culmination of everything in this book. We've reproduced the checklist here for you to reassess your new level of readiness.

Though it's written in the first person, partners can replace "I" with "she" and replace "my" with "her" to rate their beloved's readiness to ejaculate.

RATING SCALE

To complete the quiz, read each statement, close your eyes, take a deep breath, and feel how much it applies to you. Then score each sentence from 0 to 5 using this rating scale:

5 = Completely describes me all the time.

4 = Mostly describes me.

3 = Sometimes describes me.

2 = Only applies to me a little.

1 = Doesn't apply to me most of the time.

0 = Doesn't apply to me at all, or I don't know if it applies to me.

QUESTIONS

1. I love sex and am entirely proud of it.

2. My attitude is completely sex positive.

3. My mind helps me become totally aroused and romantically engaged.

4. I feel safe and trust my lover, even when my lover is me.

5. I desire to share pleasure and love in my healthy relationship, even when that's with myself.

6. I talk freely and openly about sex.

7. I can relax thoroughly during states of high arousal.

8. I totally love and accept my body and all its parts and fluids.

9. I know all the trigger points that give me the best turn-ons.

10. My tissues and erogenous zones are free and supple.

11. The sexual muscles in my pelvis are strong when I need them and relaxed otherwise.

12. I love my clitoris and know exactly how to please it.

13. I know exactly how to locate my G-spot.

14. I know exactly how to give my G-spot maximum pleasure.

15. I know how to guide a partner to give me maximum pleasure.

16. I show I'm excited by moving, breathing, making sounds, and expressing my emotions.

17. I can easily and reliably reach orgasm.

18. I have multiple, extended, and continuous full-body orgasms.

19. I know how to relax, let go, and push out to ejaculate.

20. I want to shower myself and my beloved with my feminine nectar.

GETTING STARTED

Learning to ejaculate takes patience, perseverance, and acceptance of yourself. This means to accept your level of sexual openness, and let whatever happens happen. Anticipate a lot of delightful experiments without expecting anything specific each time. Gradually, you will learn what type of stimulation works for you and when to do what. You may not become a real gusher all at once, but if you both enjoy yourselves, you'll have a fantastic time trying.

Many women may feel more comfortable trying out this new idea alone before they include a partner. If you haven't ejaculated in the past, we recommend that you begin with solo practice. Many of the taboos, pressures, and fears that can get in the way are lessened when you try it first alone.

Of course, learning solo only represents part of the story. So, later practices show you how to guide a partner to stimulate you to gushing.

FLOWING WITH INTERCOURSE

We recommend that you wait until you're confident you can ejaculate with fingers and toys before you and a male partner try it during intercourse. Getting the penis to hit the right spot with your G-spot's preferred pressure and stroke is much more of a challenge. Once you can let your waters flow, flowing during intercourse is just another step in the learning process. Another challenge during intercourse is stamina. The guy needs to be able to last long enough for the G-spot to swell and gush.

DESIGNED FOR YOUR UNIQUE ARCHITECTURE

As you know by now, reaching and playing with your own G-spot for very long can be a physical strain. Adding adequate speed and pressure to ejaculate is even more difficult.

Today, dildos come in all sizes and materials, giving you a lot to choose from. Some come with curved ends to assist you in pressuring the G-spot. Most are relatively inexpensive. As much as your budget and curiosity allow, we encourage you to try many different ones.

Some dedicated G-spot stimulators contain vibrators as well. You'll probably prefer a battery operated toy if you're planning to insert it into the vagina. If you get one, make sure it has a variable speed control to allow you to tune it to your preferred frequency.

A small vibrator with variable speed is also wonderful for simultaneous clitoris stimulation. These days you can buy a special vibrating dildo with an outside arm designed to directly excite your clitoris. Vibration inside the vagina on the G-spot and outside on the clitoris is just the ticket to ejaculation for some women.

UH, OH — THERE'S ALWAYS A CATCH

Jeffre definitely prefers having her partner stimulate her, but occasionally a change is fun. Using a sex toy can be a delightful adjunct to any sexual encounter. Having encouraged you to experiment with what turns you, whether natural, organic, or mechanical, we want to offer one critical caveat.

Don't become dependent on sex toys to squirt or have an orgasm. For all of the reasons we discussed in the healing chapter, some women seem to need extraordinarily long and hard stimulation to achieve orgasm and ejaculate. If you're one of these women, don't paint yourself into a sexual corner by only enjoying dildos and vibrators.

Besides, many sex toys look and feel good initially, but they don't live up to their sales pitch. Often, that's because of the level of sexual power and freedom of the user.

Take a lesson from our personal experience: the more deeply you explore your orgasmic potential, the more sensitive you'll become, and the less you'll need the continuously intense stimulation of vibrators. Experiment, enjoy, and expand while you keep all of your options open.

PRACTICE: SOLO EJACULATION PRACTICE

If you have a close, completely trusting relationship with someone, you may not feel the need to start by practicing alone. That's fine; you know yourself best. Even so, we encourage you to read over this practice completely before you make your final decision. The mechanics will be valuable when you start with your beloved.

By the way, here's an important reminder just in case you skipped over our earlier discussion about lubrication. Don't depend on what the vagina produces by itself. Be sure to have plenty of water-based lubricant available. It keeps the tender tissues from becoming irritated, and it means you can play longer.

Some women really like natural oils such as olive, coconut, or pure cocoa butter, but we recommend not putting oil or anything edible inside the vagina. If it's digestible, yeast and bacteria can feed upon it and throw the vagina's healthy balance out of whack. That's why we prefer water-based lubricant, particularly for inner vagina play.

PARTNERING QUESTIONS

Even for solo practices like this one, getting clear with yourself first is important. Because female ejaculation can be emotional, we offer this reminder of how to use these questions:

DESIRES: What do I want from this practice? Stay focused on your feelings, intentions, and general reasons for wanting to learn. This might be "I want to experience new sensations and practice with the new things I've learned about ejaculating." Stay away from setting goals, measurable standards, or mandatory outcomes.

CONCERNS: What are my worries or fears? Am I worried about losing control? About peeing or defecating? About not doing it "right?" How do I feel about doing this alone?

BOUNDARIES: Do I want to set up any limits or ground rules to protect myself? Are there any definite no-no's for me? Do I want to use gloves? Do I want to set a time limit?

1. PREPARE WITH THE FIVE S'S

Supplies, Showering, Setting, Stretching, and Settling. Be sure you're hydrated and have drinking water within arm's reach, as well as lots of water-based lubricant.

2. FINAL PREPARATIONS

Be sure you protect the bed or playing surface with layers of towels or protective sheeting pads. There are disposable bed protectors you can buy at your local drug store, but be sure you get the flat kind.

Empty your bladder and bowels. The confidence of knowing you're empty will help you relax. Give yourself permission to go to the toilet anytime you feel like it, however.

After all of your preparations, wash your hands again before beginning to play with yourself.

3. AWAKEN YOUR BODY

Caress and awaken your whole body softly and sensuously. Use oil on your skin if and when you choose. Begin without focusing on your most erogenous zones. Be sure to include your legs and arms, neck and face, and buttocks if it's comfortable reaching around.

Practice the four cornerstones of orgasmic breathing, and do a few PC pumps every once in awhile to stoke the sexual fires. Try brushing your inner thighs very lightly while you breathe and squeeze your PC. Then try caressing other areas that turn you on. Mix and match the sensations. It adds to the variety and the excitement.

4. APPROACH THE VAGINA

As you begin heating up, concentrate more on your erogenous zones, breasts, and vulva. Continue stimulating yourself until you're highly aroused and wet.

Move to your clitoris when you're ready. Start with gentle play, becoming firmer when you really want to. There's no rush, right?

Explore your inner lips and the vagina's mouth next. Use whatever strokes turn you on most, freely replenishing water-based lubrication as needed. As you move inside, awaken the vagina's outer section by concentrating on strokes that create delicious friction. As you move deeper into the vagina's inside area, add pressure against your vagina's walls.

Concentrate on feeling all of the sensations. What's going on where? Breathe into sensitive spots to excite them more.

5. G-SPOT

When you feel your vagina swelling, keep going. Don't rush for an orgasm, and don't try to ejaculate yet. You're still going up, up, up. Remember, without sufficient turn-on, your G-spot may remain quiet, submerged, and empty of fluid.

Now, feel around for your G-spot as you learned in the G-spot massage chapter, and focus on the strokes you learned. Use your finger(s) if that's comfortable for you, or use a G-spot wand or dildo if you prefer. It will be better if you learn how to squirt without a vibrator inside at first, if you can.

If you're aroused enough and used to it, you'll probably find G-spot play very pleasurable, but don't be alarmed if it's a neutral or somewhat uncomfortable experience at first. Your G-spot isn't an instant orgasmic trigger like your clitoris. Instead, it's a pathway that you have to travel to reach your destination.

6. EXPERIMENT

Try different body positions to learn the most convenient and direct access to your G-spot. What works best for your unique physiology? What is most comfortable for you over long periods?

Further, varying your posture, like squatting, kneeling, or getting on hands and knees, can provide different sensations and stimulation. For example, while on your back, bring your legs way up to your breasts, opening your vagina even more.

Use the four cornerstones of orgasmic breathing to energize your turn-on. In addition to deep belly breathing, moving erotically, and moaning with pleasure, squeezing your PC muscle at pivotal times can really boost your excitement.

Occasionally, relax the stimulation to your G-spot, and continue with clitoral stimulation. This can be with your fingers or even a small vibrator on the outside. Add whatever really turns you on, whether it's videos or fantasies in your mind. If you tend to be in your mind a lot in life, fantasy can help you avoid distraction and focus on the feelings in your body right now.

Then, switch back to G-spot massage for a little while. You can experiment with different rhythms, alternating between your clitoris and your G-spot. After some time, try them both together.

Reassure yourself from time to time, reminding yourself that this takes practice and relaxation. Whatever happens is okay. This isn't a race or a competition!

7. P-SIGNALS

When you get your first P-signals, your immediate reaction may be to clamp down and hold back. Don't worry about it, as that's a commonly ingrained response to the feeling that you need to urinate. Your first objective is to just let it be. Relax your whole body, breathe into the feeling, and explore the sensation. Feel the waves of pleasure and the building of desire.

If you're worried that your bladder is full again, empty it before continuing, but the truth is that you can ejaculate even when there's urine in your bladder. Most importantly, the more experience you have, the easier it will become to distinguish between the sensations of G-spot stimulation and the genuine need to urinate.

At first, we suggest you just let the sexual energy build, and resist the temptation to push the ejaculate out. You can play a little game with yourself, such as "Can I turn myself on just a little more with my breath, fantasies, fingers, and vibrator? I won't try to ejaculate until I'm just a little more turned on." You can even imagine someone playfully telling you that "you can't try just yet. You have to wait." You can only try when your imaginary master tells you it's time.

Eventually, you'll feel that your G-spot is thoroughly engorged. As you reach a peak of pleasure and feel those P-signals shooting strong rockets of sensations inside, then go for it. Push out as you slow or stop stimulation and maybe even remove your finger or toy.

If you don't squirt the first time, continue strong stroking of your G-spot until another peak and try it over and over. If it doesn't happen after a few tries, move on to the next step. If you did squirt, guess what? The advice is the same. Continue alternately stroking and pushing repeatedly.

Many women can ejaculate without a full-blown, earth-shattering orgasm. Actually, we consider every peak of pleasure to be an orgasm of sorts.

8. ORGASM

Whether or not you have ejaculated already, try it with the Big O. Using your most powerful turn-ons, including G-spot massage, stimulate yourself over the edge. As you approach orgasm, remind yourself that you know how to have an orgasm, and if that's all that happens this time, it will feel really good. All orgasms are good, right?

As your orgasm peaks, push out. This may be very new to you. In fact, you may have the urge to pull back for fear of urinating. Try to resist this impulse by reminding yourself that the bed is protected, you're safe, and there's no one else there. You can just let everything go.

If you release fluid while in the throes of orgasm, you may find that you've just had the mother of all orgasms, or you may not realize you've done it until you check underneath.

If you have the time and the inclination, you can do this all over again. Multiple orgasms and multiple ejaculations are multiply exquisite. The only limit is your physical energy, desire, and hydration. If you keep going, be sure to drink lots of water. You might want to pee again before you start the next round.

Even if you didn't ejaculate, you had a terrific orgasm, which is reason enough to celebrate. You've learned so much about your body and sensations, and if you want to ejaculate, you'll just have to practice some more. What a chore! (It sure beats cleaning the house, right?)

9. CLOSE

When you decide to end your session, relax gradually, and slow down your movements. Again, we really like the energy connection of one hand on the vagina and one hand on your heart. Reflect on what you discovered and what felt belt. Silently (or even verbally) appreciate yourself, your courage, and your strength for trying something new and exploring the pleasurable experiences of your body.

PRACTICE: PARTNER EJACULATION PRACTICE

Having a trusted partner to practice with is more fun and often more stimulating than practicing by yourself. In some ways, it's easier. You can make your body much more comfortable, and you don't need to think about so many things at once. The greatest advantage of partner play is that you can relax into the pleasure more.

Of course, you need a partner who is completely with you and on the same page. It needs to be someone who is devoted to your pleasure and willing to learn with you. You need to trust and feel safe with this person. The Partnering Questions are a vital part of this. Talk as long as you need to feel comfortable and ready to proceed.

Your partner needs to remember that every woman is different, so what may have worked for another woman may not work for you. And, as we've said, what a woman likes can vary from time to time and moment to moment.

PARTNERING QUESTIONS

DESIRES: What do each of you want from this practice? Stay focused on your feelings, intentions, and general reasons for wanting to learn. For the receiver, it might be, "I want to be relaxed enough to totally focus on my pleasure and the sensations in my body." For the giver, it might be, "I intend to be fully present and follow your directions completely." Stay away from setting goals, measurable standards, and mandatory outcomes.

CONCERNS: What are your worries or fears? Are you worried about losing control, peeing, or defecating? Are either of you worried about not doing it "right?" This includes physical, emotional, or psychological concerns about your partner's reactions. Now is a good time to talk about any medical condition or STDs that might be a factor.

BOUNDARIES: Do either of you want to set up any limits or ground rules to protect yourselves? Are there any definite no-no's or off-limit areas? Outline when and what needs to happen before penetration of any sort. Does the receiver want the giver to wear gloves?

1. PREPARE WITH THE FIVE S'S

Supplies, Showering, Setting, Stretching, and Settling.

Be sure the receiver is hydrated and that you have plenty of drinking water, as well as water-based lubricant, within arm's reach.

Discuss the Partnering Questions. Agree on any signals or alert words.

2. FINAL PREPARATIONS

Be sure you protect the bed or playing surface with layers of towels and protective sheeting pads. There are disposable bed protectors you can buy at your local drug store, but be sure you get the flat kind.

Be sure to empty your bladders and bowels. The confidence of knowing you're empty will help you relax and will prevent unnecessary interruptions. Give each other permission to go to the toilet anytime you feel like it (with warning, of course).

After all of your preparations, wash your hands again before you begin. Arrange your bodies to best reach and titillate inside the vagina. If you've completed all the practices in the G-spot massage chapter, you know what position works best for each of you. If you haven't, we suggest you refer to that chapter before you proceed.

3. AWAKEN HER BODY

If you know one another well, you know how to awaken her body. If you don't, we highly recommend the How To Touch Me Practice described in the loveplay chapter before you try this ejaculation practice.

Giver, caress and awaken the receiver's whole body slowly and sensuously, using oil if and when she chooses. There are no time limits. Begin without focusing on her most erogenous zones. Be sure to include her legs and arms, neck and face, and buttocks.

Practice the four cornerstones of orgasmic breathing, and have her perform a few PC pumps every once in awhile to stoke the sexual fires. Try brushing her inner thighs or other areas very lightly while she breathes and squeezes her PC. Mix and match sensations. It adds to the variety and the excitement.

4. APPROACH THE VAGINA

Giver, as she heats up, concentrate more on her erogenous zones. When you sense she's ready, ask permission to touch her vagina. Never make a big change without explicit permission. Approach her vagina reverently, beginning as she's previously demonstrated to you, or let her guide you entirely in the moment. Listen for her guidance, and watch for her reactions. Follow her lead at all times.

Use lots of her preferred lubricant, and continue stimulating her until she's highly aroused and wet. Move to her clitoris only when she says she's ready. Then, stimulate it exactly the way she instructs you, previously or right now. Check in with her occasionally to make sure you're doing it the way she likes. You'll probably be able to tell by her moans and sighs. Play with her clitoris and the outside of her vagina slowly and gently at first, getting firmer when she wants.

Follow her directions as she gets more and more turned on. When you notice she's very engorged, ask if she's ready for finger penetration. The choice of finger is a personal decision. Many prefer the middle finger because it's longer, while some prefer the index finger because it has maximum strength and control. Play with each of them, and let the receiver decide. Some women, as they become more swollen, actually want two or more fingers inside.

First, explore the vagina's inner lips and mouth. Use whatever strokes turn her on most, freely replenishing water-based lubrication as needed. Then, move inside, awakening the vagina's outer section with strokes that create delicious friction. As you move deeper into the inside of her vagina, add pressure against the walls.

Gently remind her to breathe, move, sound, squeeze her PC, and feel all of the sensations.

5. G-SPOT

When you feel the vagina swelling, keep going. Don't push for orgasm or ejaculation yet. She's still going up, up, up. Remember that without sufficient turn-on, her G-spot may remain quiet, submerged, and empty of fluid.

Now, find her G-spot as you learned in the sacred landscape chapter. Get confirmation from her that you're there.

Focus on G-spot massage strokes. The stroke that most women like when climbing the orgasmic ladder is the come-hither8 stroke. Remember that every woman is different, however, and each woman is different in every moment. Expect and be prepared for anything.

Though G-spot massage can be done with a dildo or vibrator, we strongly recommend you start with fingers. They're more sensitive, and you can vary the angle and pressure more easily. Besides, with fingers, the receiver will be more involved, feeling your stimulation more intimately. This allows her to give feedback and lets you react more quickly.

Eventually, you may want to move on to a sex toy just to feel the difference. Some women like firm pressure on the G-spot while using a vibrator on the clitoris. Others find that a vibrator inside and outside is the ticket to ejaculation. Remind her that there's no wrong way.

Because many women want or need very strong pressure during orgasm to ejaculate, it may require something more than fingers, but you may find that firm and fast stroking from multiple fingers works, too. Some women can even expand to receive a fist, which will frequently activate ejaculation.

Because this is a learning practice, try many things until you find just what your receiver needs and wants.

6. EXPERIMENT

Together, try different body positions to learn the most convenient and direct access to her G-spot. What works best for her unique physiology? What is most comfortable for both of you for long periods?

Further, varied postures, like squatting, kneeling, or hands and knees, can provide different sensations and stimulation. While on her back, ask her to bring her legs way up to her breasts, opening her vagina even more. The G-spot massage chapter gives further details about various positions to try.

Occasionally, relax G-spot stimulation and continue with clitoris play. This can be with your fingers or even a small vibrator on the outside. Add whatever really turns her on. Then, switch back to G-spot massage for a little while.

You can experiment with different rhythms, alternating between her clitoris and her G-spot. If you like it, excite her clitoris with your mouth, lips, and tongue. She may want more of one or the other at different times, or she may want all of them together.

You, the giver, are in total service to the receiver. She may need occasional reassurance. That's perfectly normal. You can try saying, "Let's go slow; there's no rush," "You're doing great; enjoy yourself," "I love watching you get totally turned on," "I'm having a wonderful time supporting you," "Relax; this is so much fun," or "I'm honored to explore this with you." Remind her that this takes practice and relaxation, and whatever happens is okay.

Don't forget that you're learning, too. Your reward will come when she gets it and the flood comes. Never assume you know more than she does. If you've had experience with other female ejaculators, offer your suggestions, but always let her make the decisions about how to proceed.

7. P-SIGNALS

When she gets her first P-signals, her immediate reaction may be to hold back or run to the toilet. If she wants to, let her go because it's all part of the learning. Check in with her when she returns. Was there very much urine? Does she still feel the desire even though she has urinated?

Encourage her to relax her whole body, breathe into the feelings, and explore the sensations. Feel the waves of pleasure and the building of desire. The more experience she has, the easier it will become for her to distinguish between the sensations of G-spot stimulation and the genuine need to urinate.

At first, we suggest you encourage her to just let the sexual energy build and resist the temptation to try and push ejaculate out. If you notice she is pushing out, suggest gently that she wait a bit. Remind her about PC pumps and the four cornerstones of orgasmic breathing. It's a lot to remember at first.

Eventually, when you feel her G-spot is thoroughly engorged and those P-signals are shooting strong rockets of sensations inside her, encourage her to go for it as she reaches a peak of pleasure. Signal her to push out as you slow or stop stimulation and maybe even remove your finger or toy.

If she didn't squirt the first time, continue strong stroking of her G-spot until another peak, and try it over and over. If it doesn't happen after a few tries, move on to the next step. If she did squirt, guess what? The advice is the same. Keep alternately stroking and pushing again and again.

8. ORGASM

Whether or not she ejaculated already, ask her if she wants to try it with the Big O. Using her most powerful turn-ons involving G-spot play, stimulate her continuously. Remember this most important rule when she's getting close: don't change anything. Keep the same stroke, speed, and pressure. As she approaches orgasm, continue to follow and support her process. Don't try to make her reach orgasm. When the climax starts, remind her to push out.

Be ready. Straighten your fingers, rapidly and firmly moving them in long strokes in and out. This can dramatically increase the intensity of the orgasm as well as stimulate ejaculation. Don't stop stroking until you get a clear signal from her to stop. This is important.

She may want you to stop suddenly, or she may want you to slow your stroking gradually. You may even find that she squeezes your finger or toy all the way out.

Don't worry if you don't get it exactly right this time. You can practice again after you have communicated thoroughly about what you both experienced.

We've heard some lovers at the brink of climax say things like, "Go for it," "I know you can do it," or "I really want to see you come." Unless the receiver has explicitly told you she wants this, we suggest you leave this kind of urging out of the practice. In our experience, it puts too much pressure on her.

She may release fluid while in the throes of orgasm, and she may not. Just accept whatever happens. If she wants to know what you saw or felt, tell her from a supportive place.

Another fun practice that can stimulate ejaculation in some women is spanking or slapping the vulva and clitoris with your hand. Giver, start lightly, and increase pressure as long as the receiver is giving you the green light. It's amazing how delicious this feels and how often it will trigger ejaculation, but make sure the receiver is fully aroused before you try this.

9. REPEAT

If you have the time and the inclination, you can do it all over again. Multiple orgasms and multiple ejaculations are multiply exquisite. The only limit is her physical energy, desire, and hydration. If you keep going, be sure she drinks lots of water. She might want to empty her bladder again before you start the next round.

Some multiply orgasmic women find that having two or three orgasms first helps them to get turned on enough to ejaculate. If you have a history of quick and easy multiple orgasms, give it a try. Otherwise, we don't suggest forcing it during your initial practices.

If the receiver didn't ejaculate, don't act disappointed even if you are feeling a little bit of disappointment. The two of you have just shared a beautiful orgasm. Celebrate the great time you both had together.

The first time ejaculation happens is always the hardest. It gets easier and easier, but it requires patience and practice. You are intrepid adventurers together. Act like it, and graciously accept whatever comes your way.

10. CLOSE

When she decides to end your session, gradually slow down your movements. Place one hand on her vagina and the other hand on her heart, if she likes. Talk about what you experienced, discovered, and felt. What worked best, and what didn't work?

Close your sacred space by spooning, holding each other, hugging, kissing, or whatever affectionate gestures feel good to the two of you.

PRACTICE: INTERCOURSE EJACULATION PRACTICE

For most women, ejaculation is more difficult with penis penetration. We highly recommend that the woman feel confident in her ability to ejaculate before trying to do it during intercourse. This definitely is not the time you want to be learning to ejaculate.

To understand how penis can best impact the G-spot, it will help tremendously if you thoroughly experimented with the Kama Sutra Sex Positions Chapter before doing this practice. It's not just about different postures, but focuses on how to create the kind of G-spot contact for different anatomies.

Decide together beforehand which positions, postures, and variations you want to try. Postures with the receiver's knees up against her chest may provide the best stimulation. Keep in mind that being relaxed, turned on, and releasing all expectations is as important as the position.

Caution: don't get caught up in trying 25 postures. In the beginning, agree to try two or three postures and a few variations on each. Keep your focus on pleasure, fun, and arousal. When the receiver becomes an accomplished and regular ejaculator, then you can try everything you want in one session.

1. PREPARE WITH THE FIVE S'S

Supplies, Showering, Setting, Stretching, and Settling.

Discuss the Partnering Questions. Agree on any signals or alert words.

2. FINAL PREPARATIONS

Be sure you protect the bed or playing surface with layers of towels and protective sheeting pads. Empty your bladders and bowels, and wash your hands.

Arrange your bodies to best reach and titillate inside the vagina. If you've completed all of the practices in the G-spot massage chapter, you already know what position works best for each of you. If you haven't, refer back to that chapter before proceeding.

3. LOVEPLAY

Ritually undress each other, whispering endearments and compliments as you reveal each body part. Exchange whatever loveplay turns you both on. Whatever gets her juicy and engorged and whatever gets him hard is good—extended oral sex, 69, fingers, or all of the above. There are no limits.

It's probably a good idea to get the receiver flowing with ejaculate before the giver actually enters her. The more turned on you both are, the more likely you'll be successful. If the receiver is already in the O-Zone, all of this will be easier.

4. INTERCOURSE

When the receiver is very engorged and having ejaculatory orgasms, and when the giver is plenty hard, slowly move into the first lovemaking posture you've agreed upon.

Try long, slow strokes with and without clitoris stimulation. Try short rapid strokes. Either type of strokes may stimulate ejaculation. Jeffre has found that short, rapid, and hard strokes work best some of the time, while long, slow strokes work better at other times.

Check in with each other often. Giver, ask her yes/no questions. Receiver, communicate what you need to your giver.

When she's ready, as the penis pulls back almost out of the vagina, the receiver should push out. Sometimes, she will be so into it that she will virtually push the penis all the way out with her vaginal muscles. Don't worry about that. Reinsert the penis when she stops squirting. Jeffre's experience is that not only is this motion of the penis very arousing as it comes almost all the way out, it's much easier to ejaculate when the penis isn't deep inside and pressing against her urethra.

A fun and juicy thing to do at this point is to remove the penis, and slap the vulva and clitoris. Start gently, and increase the pressure gradually. The receiver will probably start to ejaculate.

5. VARIATIONS

Experiment with variations of the first posture that you've agreed to try. As described in the positions chapter, try adjusting your leg positions and weight distribution. See which ones give the most contact between penis and G-spot. However possible within the posture, adjust for maximum G-spot stimulation. Play with different speeds, angles, pressures, and rhythms.

Remember that the goal is to stay in the state of arousal with the feelings and sensations you already know. Stay conscious of all of your senses. When the orgasmic energy is really flowing, even minor stimulation can start another ejaculation.

Pause occasionally, communicate, and enjoy, but be willing to shift when your body or partner needs a change.

Don't be afraid to bring a little bit of humor to all of this. The first time may or may not be successful. Many women who regularly ejaculate with oral sex or fingering simply can't do it with intercourse at first. So, relax, and have fun. It's all about practice.

6. NEXT POSTURE

When you agree that you've fully explored the first posture and thoroughly enjoyed all its pleasures, try one or two others in the same way. Experiment with short, long, fast, and slow strokes with and without clitoris stimulation.

7. CLOSING

When you're ready to wind down, maintain intimacy physically and emotionally. As the penis is removed, cover the vulva or each other's hearts with your hands to keep your sweet connection alive. Touch each other softly and gently. Spoon or hold each other, and synchronize your breathing.

If you want, talk briefly about what you experienced and what you'd like to try in the future. Make a date for next time. Appreciate each other for the experience, and close your sacred space with a kiss.

8. FEEDBACK

You may want to talk in greater depth later about what each of you experienced. If you do, be sure to stay focused on your own experience, and resist criticism of yourself or your partner.

FURTHER PRACTICE

Whether you, the receiver, feel you want to have further practice alone or with your partner, explore your feelings. Be honest with yourself about what you want. Some women want to squirt every time, while some women decide that ejaculation is much ado about nothing. Others become determined to learn how no matter how long it takes. Whatever you choose is a very individual decision, and there are no wrong choices.

As we said earlier, being able to ejaculate won't make you sexier, but it will give you more options for playfulness and pleasure in your sexual journey. It's truly a yummy experience, but no two women are the same.

Jeffre can ejaculate with an orgasm and without an orgasm. She can ejaculate with either G-spot stimulation or clitoris stimulation and sometimes with both. But she started not knowing how. Today, the many different sexual pleasures she enjoys are the result of curiosity, openness, and a willingness to experiment.

Sometimes, she gushes a large amount, and sometimes, it's merely a dribble. She can't predict, and she doesn't try. Interestingly, even when she doesn't let go of a large amount, it still feels as if she's releasing something. The sensations are still wonderful.

We recommend to women who want to continue practicing that they strengthen their PC muscles and enjoy self-pleasuring once or twice a week minimum. Use it or lose it definitely applies to sexuality. Intersperse your experiences with your partner with experiences alone.

The more you ejaculate, the more you will ejaculate. To some degree, it's literally a muscle that will become stronger with repetition.

ENJOY THE DELICIOUS WET JOURNEY

Whether ejaculation is for you or not, we hope you have enjoyed the journey, for there is only the journey, and pleasure rules. Remember the essential conditions mentioned earlier: relaxation, feelings of safety and acceptance, intense arousal, releasing of goals, hydration (plenty of water), surrendering to pleasure, and loving every part of yourself.

Happy ejaculating!

GLOSSARY OF TERMS

BIG O

A strong explosive orgasm.

BLENDED ORGASM

Originally, an orgasm that results from both clitoral and vaginal stimulation. We extend that definition to encompass any two or more orgasmic triggers, including orgasmic energy.

BREATH

One of the four cornerstones of supreme bliss.

BUTTERFLY

A massage stroke that uses unexpected flitting taps with your fingertips all over the body with no specific pattern.

CHANNEL ENERGY

To circulate, move, or run sexual energy throughout the body.

CERVIX

The lower end or neck of the uterus which opens into the top end of the vagina.

CHAKRA

One of seven centers inside the body from the bottom of the spine to the top of the head where subtle energy is generated, collected, stored, and swirled. Though energy is energy, it has different qualities at each chakra.

CHI

See Energy.

CLITORIS

A highly-sensitive sexual organ. Its head lies under the intersection of a woman's inner lips and also has "legs" which extend deeper toward the sides of the vagina.

COME-HITHER

A G-spot massage stroke which involves crooking one or more fingers back toward your palm as if you were beckoning someone to come toward you.

CORNERSTONES

Four simple but powerful physical skills used to generate ecstasy at will—presence (relaxation, mental focus, and concentration), breath, sound, and movement.

CRURA

The legs of the clitoris which extend deeper inside a woman's body on either side of the vagina.

EJACULATE

To push out sperm or female ejaculate liquid.

ENERGY

The nervous stimulation and physical excitation that our bodies feel all the time, which is responsible for emotional sensations and the physical manifestation of the spirit. Most strongly felt by most as a result of sexual stimulation and orgasm.

ENGORGED

When sensitive organs composed of erectile tissue swell with blood and darken from arousal.

ERECTILE TISSUE

The technical name for sensitive organs that swell with blood and darken when aroused, also known as engorgement.

EROGENOUS ZONES

Parts of the body that arouse sexual desire when you touch them.

EXPLOSIVE ORGASM

The kind of sudden strong orgasm that relieves tension and releases energy quickly in a flash of pleasure, which is accompanied by ejaculation in men and often drains lovers of their energy.

FEEDBACK SANDWICH

A diplomatic way that lovers can ask for changes in sexual play or other behavior without hurting their partner's feelings. The feedback sandwich is a communication cycle, beginning and ending with positive reinforcement, which begins with a compliment, asks for something different, and finally acknowledges what's working.

FEMALE PROSTATE

Spongy erectile tissue made up of a series of small paraurethral glands and ducts surrounding the urethra along the roof of the vagina. *See* G-spot, Paraurethral Glands, Urethral Sponge, Skene's Glands.

FOUR CORNERSTONES OF SUPREME BLISS

Breath, sound, movement, and presence.

FULL-BODY ORGASM

An energetic implosive orgasm throughout the entire body accompanied by writhing, undulating, and vibrating all over as a result of channeling sexual energy out of the genitals. *See* Implosive Orgasm.

GLANS

The rounded tip of the clitoris or penis.

G-SPOT

A small, mobile pleasure point usually located a few inches deep on the upper part of the vaginal channel, first reported in the 1950s by the gynecologist, Dr. Ernst Gräfenberg, as the female orgasmic trigger. *See* Female Prostate, Paraurethral Glands, Urethral Sponge, Skene's Glands.

HOT SPOTS

Tissues inside the vagina that need healing. She may feel tension, numbness, tenderness, soreness, pain, burning, or a bruised feeling in these areas.

IMPLOSIVE ORGASM

A long series of slow, pleasurable vibrations in both men and women accompanied with a rush of orgasmic energy which occurs when sexual arousal gets pumped back inside and is circulated over and over again without explosive release.

INNER FLUTE

The invisible channel near the spine that connects the chakras. *See* Chakras.

KEGELS

Exercises originally developed by a gynecologist named Dr. Arnold Kegel in 1952 to teach women to regain control of their urinary reflexes by restoring tone to their PC muscles after the trauma of childbirth. *See* PC Muscle.

KUNDALINI

Loosely, sexual or orgasmic energy. The normally latent psychosexual power, likened to a coiled snake, that lies dormant at the base of the spine. When awakened, Kundalini energy can ascend through the subtle body, creating powerful ecstatic experiences and heightened cosmic consciousness. *See* Energy.

LOVEPLAY
Any kind of intimate, physical, sexual frolicking that creates turn-on and demonstrates love, affection, and desire. Foreplay is included, but loveplay extends throughout the lovemaking experience, not just as a precursor to intercourse and can even be an end in itself.

MEDITATION
Sitting and emptying the mind by reciting mantras, watching the breath, or witnessing ideas floating by, intended to create a "no mind" condition of deep inner peace filled with stillness.

MOVE ENERGY
To circulate, channel, or run sexual energy throughout the body.

ORGASM
Sexual climax, the moment of most intense pleasure in sexual stimulation, usually accompanied with explosive release, and sometimes by an unlimited, timeless, whole body-mind-spirit altered state.

ORGASMIC BREATHING
The kind of breath, sound, movement, and presence that happens when you have a typical exciting explosive orgasm. Consciously and intensely using these four cornerstones will heighten sexual ecstasy. *See* Four Cornerstones of Supreme Bliss.

ORGASMIC ENERGY
Strong, pleasurable sensations and energy accompanied by intense sexual arousal.

O-ZONE OR ORGASM ZONE
The high plateau of sexual ecstasy where you float continuously with multiple and lengthy full-body mind-blowing energetic orgasms.

PARAURETHRAL GLANDS
A collection of up to 40 small glands, accompanied by ducts and blood vessels, surrounding the female urethra along the roof of the vagina. Also known as Urethral Sponge, G-spot, Female Prostate, and Skene's Glands.

PC MUSCLE
Short for pubococcygeus. The muscle that snakes down around the anus and genitals connecting the pubic bone to the coccyx bones plus the sitting bones and legs.

PEAK

Letting sexual excitement rise to a high level and then, immediately drop back down, which, if graphed, looks like scaling a steep mountain peak followed by a precipitous fall.

PEAKING

Adjusting the sexual stimuli that cause sudden surges of arousal in order to come back down without going over the top to orgasm.

PERINEUM

The general region of the pelvic floor between the genitals and the anus.

PLATEAU

An ongoing high level of sexual arousal that continues without diminishing.

PLEASURE BALLOON

An energy bubble that is imagined inside, which limits and controls your capacity to feel. At rest, your pleasure balloon is collapsed around your genitals. As you become excited and filled with orgasmic energy, your balloon expands.

PRE-ORGASMIC

Referring to a woman who hasn't yet experienced an orgasm.

PRESENCE

One of the four cornerstones of supreme bliss, which means to relax enough to open your senses in the moment without any goal or expectation and with 100% focus on the pleasure you feeling right now.

P-SIGNAL

The sensation of a swelling G-spot that initially feels like the need to urinate but which actually signals the right time for a woman to push out, expel fluid, and ejaculate.

PUBOCOCCYGEUS

See PC Muscle.

SACRED SPACE

Consciously making the environment in which you explore your sexuality a special place. This includes cleaning and beautifying the room you choose.

S.E.X.

Subtle Energy eXchange. Any touching, moving, meditating, or erotic sharing, including fantasy, which stimulates and connects lovers' inner vibrations.

SELF-PLEASURING

A term for masturbation during which one honors one's body and celebrates pleasure.

SEX POSITIVE
An attitude and mindset in which you know that sexual ecstasy is good for you.

SIGNALS
Words, sounds, or hand motions used to give feedback to a sexual partner about erotic reactions and arousal level.

SKENE'S GLANDS
Another name for the spongy erectile tissue made up of a series of many small glands and ducts surrounding the urethra along the roof of the vagina. Named after Alexander Skene, M.D., who studied and drew them in great detail in 1880. *See* G-spot, Female Prostate, Paraurethral Glands, Urethral Sponge.

STREAMING
To circulate, move, run, or channel sexual energy, often without sexual stimulation, to create strong pleasurable spasms and energetic vibrations.

URETHRA
The tube or canal through which urine is discharged in both men and women.

URETHRAL SPONGE
Spongy erectile tissue made up of a series of up to 40 small paraurethral glands and ducts surrounding the urethra along the roof of the vagina. *See* G-spot, Female Prostate, Skene's Glands, Paraurethral Glands.

UTERUS
A pear-shaped, hollow muscular organ or womb in which a fertilized egg grows into an embryo, fetus, and baby.

YAB-YUM
The paramount sexual position named for the Buddhist term "union of mother and father" in which the man sits cross-legged with the woman on his lap with her legs wrapped around him.

OTHER AMORATA PRESS BOOKS

MALE MULTIPLE ORGASM: TECHNIQUES THAT GUARANTEE YOU AND YOUR LOVER INTENSE SEXUAL PLEASURE AGAIN AND AGAIN AND AGAIN
Somraj Pokras, $13.95
This book teaches a man how to make love for hours while giving his partner absolute pleasure again and again.

EROTIC MASSAGE FOR LOVERS: SENSUAL TOUCH FOR INTIMACY AND ORGASMIC PLEASURE
Rosalind Widdowson & Steve Marriott, $16.95
Designed to help lovers unleash the dynamic potential of the erogenous zones all over the body, this book explores a range of sexually charged movements and manipulations, with some surprising additions and ingenious variations.

THE LITTLE BIT NAUGHTY BOOK OF SEX POSITIONS
Siobhan Kelly, $11.95
Fully illustrated with 50 tastefully explicit color photos, *The Little Bit Naughty Book of Sex Positions* provides everything readers need to start using these thrilling new positions tonight.

ORGASMS: A SENSUAL GUIDE TO FEMALE ECSTASY

Nicci Talbot, $16.95

Straight-talking and informative, *Orgasms* is a girl's best friend when it comes to understanding the physical, psychological, and spiritual factors contributing to great sex and intense orgasms.

ORGASM EVERY DAY EVERY WAY EVERY TIME: A WOMAN'S GUIDE TO SEXUAL PLEASURE

Jenny Wood, $12.95

Dishes up everything from fantastic foreplay tips and mind-blowing masturbation techniques to orgasm-inducing intercourse positions and creative new ways to reach that peak of ecstasy.

UNLEASHING HER G-SPOT ORGASM: A STEP-BY-STEP GUIDE TO GIVING A WOMAN ULTIMATE SEXUAL ECSTASY

Donald L. Hicks, $12.95

Drawing on the latest findings of world-reknowned sex researchers, this useful handbook offers a unique combination of clinical fact and everyday application.

THE WILD GUIDE TO SEX AND LOVING

Siobhan Kelly, $16.95

Packed with practical, frank and sometimes downright dirty tips on how to hone your bedroom skills, this handbook tells you everything you need to know to unlock the secrets of truly tantalizing sensual play.

To order these books call 800-377-2542 or 510-601-8301, fax 510-601-8307, e-mail ulysses@ulyssespress.com, or write to Amorata Press, P.O. Box 3440, Berkeley, CA 94703. All retail orders are shipped free of charge. California residents must include sales tax. Allow two to three weeks for delivery.

ABOUT THE AUTHORS

SOMRAJ POKRAS is the author of *Male Multiple Orgasm* and many books on Tantra and Tantric Sex, as well as the leader of 50 people skills workshops. As co-founder of TantraAtTahoe.com, he's written hundreds of informative web pages and how-to articles as part of publishing their free weekly newsletter. During his 35-year career as a counselor, group facilitator, and trainer, Somraj has guided more than 20,000 people to lead more effective lives. He derives great joy from assisting others to release inhibitions that block their pleasure so they can enjoy life, love, and ecstatic lovemaking for hours and hours.

DR. JEFFRE TALLTREES is a psychologist, sex therapist, shaman and senior staff member of The Four Winds Society, an international school of shamanic healing. She is a columnist and author, co-authoring *Hotter Sex Deeper Love*, *Tantric G-Spot Orgasm* and *Supreme Bliss Tantric Guide for Couples*. Dr. TallTrees is a Tantric master and co-founder of Tantra At Tahoe, where she teaches couples ways to improve their intimacy and their lovelife.